The Source for Down Syndrome

Catherine E. Chamberlain

Robin M. Strode

D1613498

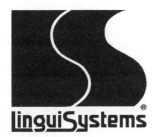

LinguiSystems

LinguiSystems, Inc.
3100 4th Avenue
East Moline, IL 61244-9700
1-800 PRO IDEA
1-800-776-4332

FAX: 1-800-577-4555
E-mail: service@linguisystems.com
Web: www.linguisystems.com
TDD: 1-800-933-8331
(for the hearing impaired)

Printed in the U.S.A.

ISBN 0-7606-0352-9

About the Authors

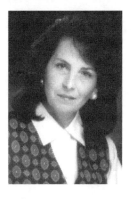

Catherine E. Chamberlain, M.A., CCC-SLP, has had over 28 years experience as a speech-language pathologist. She maintains a private practice serving the preschool population. Catherine also works at the Early Childhood Development Center in Winchester, Kentucky and she formerly worked in the public schools for 14 years. She has special interest in working with students with autism, Down syndrome, and multiple handicaps.

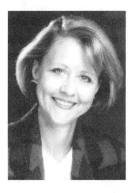

Robin M. Strode, M.A., CCC-SLP, has had over 26 years experience as a speech-language pathologist. She has been in private practice for over 18 years. In addition to her private practice, Robin works at the Early Childhood Development Center in Winchester, Kentucky. She has also worked as a part-time instructor in the Communication Disorders Department at the University of Kentucky. Prior to entering private practice, Robin worked in the public schools for eight years. She has special interest in working with students with developmental delays, autism, Down syndrome, developmental verbal apraxia, oral-motor issues, speech/phonological disorders, and language disorders.

Catherine and Robin have served as consultants to speech-language pathologists, teachers, schools, and families. They have presented numerous workshops on apraxia and oral-motor skills throughout the country. *The Source for Down Syndrome* is their sixth joint publication for LinguiSystems. They have also written *Easy Does It for Apraxia and Motor Planning; Easy Does It for Apraxia – Preschool; Easy Does It for Articulation: An Oral-Motor Approach; Easy Does It for Voice;* and *SPARC for Concepts.* Catherine is also the author of *Best Concept Workbook Ever* and *Best Concept Pictures Ever.*

Dedications/Acknowledgments

To the parents, siblings, teachers, therapists, extended families, and friends of the children and adults with Down syndrome who provide support, encouragement, and love to help them attain their goals and to enjoy interesting and productive lives. And as always, to my home team, who are always behind me 100%. — CC

To the great teachers who have inspired us to be better than we thought we could be: Dr. Robert Mason, Dr. William Durbin, and Terry Johnson. And as always, to my greatest supporters: Tom, Cole, Harry Miller, and W.Q. Stacy. — RS

Illustrations by Margaret Warner and Ken Prestley
Cover Design by Mike Paustian
Page Layout by Christine Buysse

Table of Contents

Table of Contents, *continued*

Introduction

The Source for Down Syndrome is written primarily to describe communication development and intervention for the child and adolescent with Down syndrome. This book addresses specific areas of development:

- feeding and oral-motor skills
- motor and sensorimotor skills
- language
- speech

However, all areas of development are interrelated and it is impossible to plan intervention without first understanding the impact of Down syndrome on the whole child and on all of his or her areas of development. Deficits or strengths in one area can have a significant impact on other areas. For example, communication skills are greatly influenced by the child's cognitive, processing, and sensori-motor systems.

Physical appearance and learning abilities can be similar in the Down syndrome population due to anatomic and physiologic differences in the brain and the body, but it is important to remember that each individual with Down syndrome is unique with his or her own personality, strengths, weaknesses, differences, and interests.

Working with individuals with Down syndrome is a truly rewarding experience. We hope you love working with these children and adolescents as much as we do. We learn so much from them every day and they bring such joy to our hearts.

Catherine and Robin

"If you treat an individual as he is, he will stay as he is; but if you treat him as if he were what he ought to be and could be, he will become what he ought to be and could be."

— Goethe

It Matters To This One

As I walked along the seashore,
This young boy greeted me.
He was tossing a stranded starfish
Back into the deep blue sea.
I said, "Tell me why you bother.
Why waste your time this way?
There are a million stranded starfish.
Does it matter anyway?"

And he said, "It matters to this one.
It deserves a chance to grow.
It matters to this one.
I can't save them all, I know.
But it matters to this one,
I'll return it to the sea.
It matters to this one,
And it matters a lot to me."

As I walked into a classroom,
The teacher greeted me.
She was helping Johnny study.
He was struggling, I could see.
I said, "Tell me why you bother.
Why waste your time this way?
Johnny's only one of millions.
Does it matter anyway?"

And she said, "It matters to this one.
He deserves a chance to grow.
It matters to this one.
I can't save them all, I know.
But it matters to this one,
I'll help him be what he can be.
It matters to this one,
And it matters a lot to me."

Author Unknown

Chapter 1: Definition, Types, and Causes of Down Syndrome

Down syndrome is the most common genetic cause of developmental disabilities. It is the result of a chromosomal disorder that causes physical and cognitive differences. Individuals with Down syndrome have three number 21 chromosomes instead of two in some or all cells. Individuals with Down syndrome manifest a range of characteristics, with some individuals presenting most of the characteristics of the syndrome and others presenting only a few. Down syndrome is found in all racial and ethnic groups. Down syndrome occurs in 1 in 800–1000 births. There are approximately 5000 children born with Down syndrome each year. Following are some common questions and answers about Down syndrome.

What are the main characteristics of children with Down syndrome?

- distinctive facial, brain, and skeletal features
- short stature
- low muscle tone
- mental retardation
- cognitive dysfunction

Are there different types of Down syndrome?

There are three types of Down syndrome: Trisomy 21, Translocation, and Mosaicism.

Humans have 50,000 — 100,000 genes. Typically, all cells have 23 pairs of chromosomes. Chromosome #21 has about 1.7% of the genetic material, or an estimated 850 to 1700 genes.

Trisomy 21 is the most common type of Down syndrome, comprising 95% of occurrences. In this type, there is an extra 21st chromosome, with each cell having 47 rather than 46 chromosomes. It results from an accident in cell division during the production of the egg or sperm cell. Five percent of children with *Trisomy 21* receive the extra 21st chromosome from the father and 95% receive the extra chromosome from the mother.

Translocation makes up approximately 4 to 5% of Down syndrome occurrences. In this type, the extra 21st chromosome becomes attached to or incorporated into another chromosome in every cell, usually chromosome 14, 21, or 22. It may occur spontaneously or may be inherited from one parent. If one parent is a carrier, there is an increased risk of other children having Down syndrome.

Mosaicism is the least common type of Down syndrome, comprising approximately 1% of occurrences. In this type, some cells have an extra chromosome (i.e., 47) and others have the normal number of chromosomes (i.e., 46). Because only certain cells are involved, the child may be less affected cognitively and physically. This type of Down syndrome is caused by an accident in cell division in the developing embryo and is thought to be due to an error in one of the first cell divisions shortly after conception.

What causes Down syndrome?

Down syndrome is a chromosome abnormality that occurs at conception or during initial cell divisions in the embryo. The cause is unknown, but there may be some relation to:

- genetics
- exposure to X-rays
- viral infections
- certain potent drugs
- hormonal and immunological problems
- maternal age
- paternal age

Is Down syndrome related to parental age?

Eighty percent are born to mothers under the age of 35. Increased maternal age increases the risk of having a child with Down syndrome from 1 in 400 at age 35 to 1 in 110 at age 40. There may also be a relationship with paternal age, but this has not been well established. In approximately 20-30% of cases, the extra 21st chromosome comes from the father.

What is the impact of Down syndrome?

As a result of having an extra 21st chromosome, the child may have structural and functional abnormalities throughout his body and the central nervous system. These may affect neurologic and cognitive functioning, health, body and organ structure and function, motor skills, muscle tone, communication skills, developmental skills, and learning.

How is Down syndrome diagnosed?

It is diagnosed by a chromosome analysis soon after birth. This karyotyping also determines the type of Down syndrome. Down syndrome can also be identified before birth through prenatal testing.

Do all people with Down syndrome have mental retardation?

Yes. The I.Q. falls mostly in the mild to moderately retarded range, although some individuals function in the near-normal range and others fall in the severely retarded range.

Chapter 2: Characteristics Found in Down Syndrome

The child with Down syndrome has unique physical, neurological, musculoskeletal, sensorimotor, learning, and communication characteristics that can impact each other as well as impact the child's ability to develop age-appropriate skills. Individuals with Down syndrome may demonstrate some or all of the following characteristics.

Physical Characteristics/Body Features

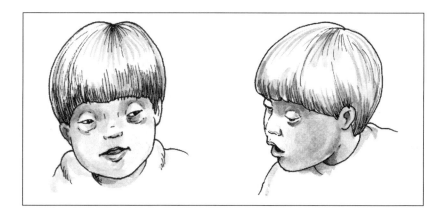

Skull   Typically, the skull is small with a shortened anterior-posterior diameter. There is rarely true microcephaly, but 80% have a head circumference that is below normal.

Midface   Typically, there is hypoplasia of the midfacial bones with reduced or increased distance between the eyes, a depressed nasal bridge, and an underdeveloped maxilla. This results in a rather flat facial appearance in the young child. The sinuses are underdeveloped and the mandible may be underdeveloped with the mandibular angle being somewhat obtuse. This can result in malocclusion and a protrusive jaw.

maxilla

mandible

mandibular angle

Eyes   Approximately 1/4 to 3/4 of children with Down syndrome are born with epicanthal folds. These small skin folds on the inner corner of the eyes are usually bilateral and may be prominent at birth. With growth of the nasal bones, the folds may disappear or become less apparent as the nasal bone pulls the adjacent skin laterally.

Oblique palpebral fissures (i.e., grooves that separate the upper and lower eyelids) are present over 95% of the time. These narrow grooves may slant upward.

The child typically has oval-shaped eyes and may have hyper- or hypotelorism (i.e., wide or narrowly-spaced eyes).

Seventy-five percent of children with Down syndrome have Brushfield spots (i.e., fine white spots in the periphery of the iris). These may not be noted in the newborn. They are seen more often in children with lighter-colored irises.

Nose/
Nasopharynx The nose tends to be small with a flat nasal bridge. At birth, the nasal bones are underdeveloped and not ossified which makes the midface look flat. Deviation of the nasal septum is common, and there tends to be underdevelopment of the frontal and paranasal sinuses.

The nasopharynx may be small due to the shape of the skull. Nasal obstruction is common.

Ears The ears tend to be significantly affected with possible abnormal structure found in the external, middle, and/or inner ears.

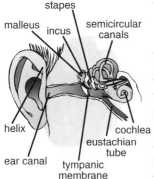

The external ear tends to be small and shortened. It is common to see an overlapping or a folding of the helix (i.e., the outer portion of the ear). One or both ears may be set low and obliquely. There is often a prominent antihelix, absent or attached earlobes, and/or projecting ears.

The middle ear may have a small, narrow ear canal; abnormalities of the tympanic membrane; poor development of mastoid air cells; and ossicular abnormalities. The middle ear bones can become eroded as a result of chronic inflammation from infection and fluid. There is a tendency toward eustachian tube dysfunction due

to an abnormal positioning in the nasopharynx and differences in tube firmness. There is also a tendency toward ear wax buildup.

There are often congenital abnormalities of the inner ear involving the cochlea, the posterior semicircular canal, and other structures.

Mouth/
Pharynx The oral cavity is small, particularly in relation to the tongue size. The palate is narrow and high arched and/or short. A bifid uvula or cleft may be present.

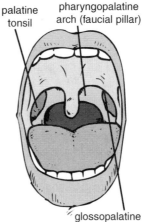

The oral pharynx tends to be small. The small oral cavity and the narrowing of the pharynx at the faucial pillars result in a superior positioning of the tonsils, which may then contribute to a pattern of tongue protrusion. The tonsils and adenoids may be large, or large in comparison to the pharynx.

The child's generalized hypotonia contributes to tongue protrusion, decreased lip closure, and poor jaw stability which allows the jaw to drop and the tongue to come forward. The hypotonia also contributes to an immature swallowing pattern. The child's pattern of mouth breathing may be secondary to enlarged adenoids/tonsils and a small oronasal pharynx along with recurrent allergies or colds.

Lips The lips appear normal in infancy, but they tend to become more prominent, thickened, and fissured over time. This is related to an habitual open-mouth posture, mouth breathing, tongue protrusion, and excessive moisture on the lips.

Tongue As a newborn, the tongue is smooth and normal in texture. As the child grows, she begins to develop papillary enlargement and fissuring (i.e., splitting) of the tongue which is thought to be due to excessive sucking or chewing of the tongue. The tongue is furrowed in 59% of individuals with Down syndrome. Hypotonia of the tongue with protrusive lips and an open-mouth posture is common.

About 57 to 75% of individuals with Down syndrome actually have an enlarged tongue; others just seem to be enlarged because of the relatively small oral cavity and underdeveloped maxilla.

Teeth/ Occlusion Malocclusion is common due to an underdevelopment of the maxilla and/or protrusion of the mandible and functional anomalies of the tongue and oral musculature. Types of occlusion anomalies noted are crossbite, protrusive mandible, excessive frontal overbite, inversion of the front teeth, and poor alignment of the teeth during occlusion so that only a few teeth meet during chewing. In addition, because of facial skeletal abnormalities, there is a change in the functional abilities of the facial muscles so that the jaw often does not open, close, and grade efficiently.

Both sets of teeth erupt one to two years later than typically-developing children and the sequence of eruption often is different. Permanent teeth may be small. There is a high incidence of peg-shaped incisors; slender, pointed canines; and congenitally missing teeth.

The child with Down syndrome has a lower prevalence of cavities than typically-developing children. However, almost all have periodontal disease which may be due to low resistance secondary to immuno-deficiency. Some other factors may be poor blood circulation, differences in connective tissue, disorders of collagen maturation, and difficulty absorbing vitamin A.

Neck The newborn may present a short, broad neck with loose skin at the nape that becomes less apparent as the child grows. The base of the neck stays broad as the child ages. The neck usually has a full range of motion.

Larynx The child may have anatomical abnormalities including a narrowing of the airway below the vocal folds (subglottic stenosis). This is usually a mild to moderate stenosis, but may be aggravated by intubation during surgeries to correct heart or gastrointestinal abnormalities. In addition, hypotonia may affect muscle tone and tension of the vocal folds.

Chest The chest usually has a normal shape although the rib cage may look shortened. There may be 11 instead of 12 ribs, or a rudimentary twelfth rib. There may be some deformities of the sternum, but these do not interfere with respiratory or cardiovascular functions.

Heart Approximately 40% of children with Down syndrome have congenital heart disease or defects. This is the most potentially serious health problem in newborns. Fifty percent of children with Trisomy 21 have congenital heart malformations which are the main cause of death in the first two years of life. It is found more often in females than in males. One or more defects may be present.

The major complications of heart defects are pulmonary artery hypertension (i.e., constriction of the blood vessels in the lungs) and pulmonary vascular obstructive disease in association with congestive heart failure. It is important to recognize and treat cardiac problems early in life before pulmonary complications become irreversible.

It may be difficult to recognize cardiac problems in the newborn child with Down syndrome because signs may not be apparent at birth; however, this can change significantly during the first few weeks of life.

The infant and child with heart defects may demonstrate increased irritability and reduced endurance and energy. Adults with Down syndrome may have an enlarged partition between the ventricles of the heart, and may demonstrate a high frequency of aortic regurgitation (i.e., blood flow from the aorta back into the left ventricle) and asymptomatic mitral valve prolapse (i.e., incomplete closure of the valve between the left atrium and ventricle). It is important that individuals with these conditions have a course of antibiotics before dental or surgical procedures to decrease the chances of heart infection.

Abdomen There is reduced muscle tone in the abdomen which often is distended and protuberant in the young child. Umbilical hernias are fairly common.

Gastro-intestinal Children with Down syndrome have an increased incidence of constipation, feeding problems, intestinal obstructions, and failure to thrive. Approximately 12% of them have congenital gastrointestinal malformations. The most common malformations include pyloric stenosis, fistulas between the trachea and esophagus causing food or liquid to be aspirated into the lungs, duodenal obstructions, absence of the anal opening, and Hirschsprung's Disease (i.e., absence of nerve cells in the rectum and colon that stimulate intestinal mobility).

Extremities There are shortened bones throughout the body. Typically, hands and feet are short, broad, and stubby. About 50% of individuals with Down syndrome have abnormally short fingers or toes and/or abnormal bending of one or more fingers or toes. Some individuals have partial or complete webbing or fusion of the fingers or toes.

The single transverse palmar crease of the hand (i.e., the straight line across the palm of hand), seen as a common trait, actually

occurs in only about 1/2 to 2/3 of children with Down syndrome.

Musculo-skeletal Characteristic of the child with Down syndrome is low muscle tone, muscle weakness, and excessive joint flexibility.

Low muscle tone generally affects all of the muscles, although the degree of low tone varies from child to child. There can be lower tone in certain parts of the body than in others. Muscle weakness may be secondary to low muscle tone and/or heart problems.

In the newborn, the muscles typically are floppy and flaccid and the child may move less. As the child develops, low tone slows the rate at which she learns major motor skills. She is later in achieving head control, feeding skills, sitting, standing, walking, and speech skills. Low tone also affects respiration and breath support for speech. Muscle tone usually improves with age.

Excessive joint flexibility is due to deviations in the collagenous connective tissue. This results in laxity of ligaments, tendons, and joint capsules. It leads to hyperflexibility and hyperextension of joints, both of which can affect motor development by reducing stability of the musculoskeletal system.

Spine There is increased incidence of intervertebral disease and degenerative arthritis of the cervical vertebrae. There may be stiffening of the lower cervical vertebral joints.

Scoliosis, or curvature of the spine, can be a serious orthopedic problem in individuals with Down syndrome. It may be caused by poor posture, poor muscle tone, and/or ligamentous laxity. It typically occurs in the thoracolumbar region and usually is mild. Severe scoliosis can cause cardiopulmonary failure.

Another serious orthopedic problem seen in 10-30% of those with Down syndrome is atlantoaxial instability. In this condition, there is an abnormal increase in joint mobility between the first two cervical vertebra. This results in differences in spacing of the cervical vertebrae that can cause compression of the spinal cord. It typically is due to anomalies in the upper cervical vertebrae and ligament laxity.

Hips   There can be some instability of the hips due to laxity of the tissues and joints. There may be spontaneous dislocation of the hip which is evidenced by a sudden onset of a limp or a reluctance to bear weight.

Knees   Instability of the knee is more common than hip instability. Difficulties range from partial dislocation of the knee with no symptoms to a complete severe dislocation.

Feet   About 90% of individuals with Down syndrome have foot deformities such as flat feet secondary to ligamentous laxity. A wide-based gait and a tendency to rotate the foot and ankle outward contribute to pronation and collapse of the midfoot.

Neurology of the Brain

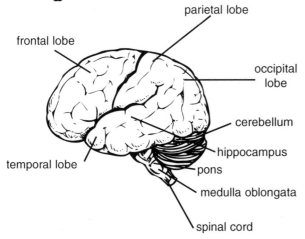

The brain of the individual with Down syndrome exhibits alterations in the shape, size, development, and function that result in mild to moderate neuropsychological impairments.

For children with Down syndrome, the shape of the brain and its size does not differ significantly from that of other children at birth. However, starting at three to six months, brain size begins to drop below normal, and important differences are observed by six months of age.

After six months of age, the brain of the child with Down syndrome is usually smaller than her peers, although 20% of those with Down syndrome have brains that remain in the lower normal range. The predominant difference is a shorter length in the anterior-posterior dimension. This includes reduction or hypoplasia of the frontal lobes and flattening of the occipital lobes. The occipitofrontal circumference typically is more than two standard deviations below normal.

Central nervous system changes accelerate during late infancy and early childhood. By late infancy, brain development slows and matures less rapidly and extensively. After mid-infancy, brain weight is usually 10-50% less than that of same age peers. By the age of three, 50% of children with Down syndrome have head circumferences that are smaller than their peers. This is true of 80% of children with Down syndrome by age five. The decreased brain weight in Down syndrome infants parallels their small heads.

The cerebral cortex is the most affected region of the brain in Down syndrome. There is a significant reduction in the total number of neurons, dendritic spines, and synaptic connections (i.e., the functional connections between neurons) in the cortex. The average length of synapses is diminished, an occurrence which increases with age. This results in deficiencies in synaptic transmissions and an impoverished dendritic environment, both of which can impact the efficiency and smoothness of transmissions as well as the integrated functioning of the neurological system. The effect is found more in the posterior brain and in the left hemisphere, rather than in the right.

There is a reduction of the density of neurons in several areas of the cerebral cortex in 10-50% of individuals with Down syndrome, which results in a smaller brain size. The impact of this decrease in neurons is loss of specific cell arrangements responsible for providing distinct boundaries between the cortical areas. This results in deficiencies in the intercorrelation between the lobes of the brain. These problems are most commonly found in the primary and associative areas (found in all lobes of the brain), the frontal cortex, the hippocampus, and the cerebellum.

One-quarter of children with Down syndrome may have a delay of myelin formation in the nervous system which mainly affects the associated and intercortical fibers of the frontal lobes, the temporal lobes, and the association cortex. There appear to be differences in the neuro-transmitter system, which may account for the differences in the reactivity (i.e., slowness to react and respond) to the environment found in those with Down syndrome.

There is unilateral or bilateral narrowing of the superior temporal gyrus in 1/3 to 1/2 of those with Down syndrome as they get older. It is two times as likely to be narrow in the left cerebral hemisphere. There tend to be more speech abnormalities in those who have narrowing of the superior temporal gyrus bilaterally or in the dominant hemisphere.

The cerebellum and brainstem are often small and weigh disproportionately less in comparison to the cerebrum. There also may be decreased development of some structures such as the secondary gyri, the corpus callosum, and the anterior commissure (which forms connections between the brain hemispheres), and the hippocampus.

There may be a relationship between the neural abnormalities and other problems in Down syndrome such as congenital heart disease and a delayed or an aberrant auditory system that may contribute to hearing disorders.

Seizure activity is noted in a small number of individuals with Down syndrome. The most common type in infants is infantile spasms followed by tonic-clonic convulsions. Some of these increase with age, which is opposite of what is found in the typical population. Tonic-clonic seizures, partial simple seizures, and partial complex seizures are the types most noted as children with Down syndrome grow older. This pattern of seizure is not solely due to abnormal brain development, but also to complicating factors such as respiratory distress, hypoxia, cardiac disease, and infections.

Neuropathological changes are seen early in life and become more prominent and prevalent by early adolescence. Young adults show smaller brains and intracranial volume than their peers.

After the age of 35, neuropathology resembling Alzheimer's Disease (AD) is common in Down syndrome. Nearly all adults with Down syndrome show neuropathology similar to that associated with AD, but less than 50% show the dementia characteristic of AD. Actually, there seems to be an extended period of asymptomatic brain disease, delaying the onset of dementia. The most prominent changes are found in the hippocampus, the temporal lobe, and the cerebellum.

In summary, individuals with Down syndrome have central nervous dysfunction secondary to abnormal brain development at all stages of brain maturation. This includes:

- reduction in the weight of the brain hemispheres, the brain stem, and the cerebellum
- delay in myelinization
- reduction in the number of neurons in the whole cerebral cortex, but more in some cortical layers
- reduction in synaptic density and functioning

The pattern of abnormal brain development in Down syndrome most likely reflects genetically-determined, altered brain programming. The neural dysfunctions in Down syndrome are not spread evenly throughout the brain, but affect some parts more than others. For example, the medial temporal lobe, particularly the hippocampus, is more often affected. It is involved in spatial cognition, flexible learning, the consolidation of what has already been learned, and retention of skills, all of which are difficult for the individual with Down syndrome.

The cerebellum is also affected. It is thought to be involved in motor skills and in acquisition of conditioned responses, areas that are impaired in persons with Down syndrome.

Reduced attention and vigilance, increased distractibility, and difficulty maintaining performance of a task are behaviors commonly found in individuals with Down syndrome. These behaviors can be related to dysfunction in the pre-frontal cortex which is important for initiation and guidance of behaviors.

There is a correlation between brain pathology and cognitive behavior in Down syndrome. The brain uses multiple learning/memory systems, some of which are more affected than others. Individuals with Down syndrome usually have greater language difficulties than other individuals with similar levels of retardation. Individuals with Down syndrome have:

- difficulty processing, retaining, and retrieving visual and especially auditory information
- reduced short-term memory
- increased difficulty recalling sequences of information
- reduced decision-making ability
- difficulty retaining information and programming sequences of behavior, both of which are frontal lobe activities

Motor Skills

Significant deficits in motor skills are common in individuals with Down syndrome. Typically these deficits are structural, sensory, and neuromotor based. Specifically, shortened bones, instability of the vertebrae of the neck, heart defects, low tone, muscle weakness, excessive joint flexibility, laxity of ligaments/tendons/ joints, and deficits in postural control all affect motor development. There often are delays in acquisition of motor milestones and a decrease in the quality of movements, including oral-motor movements. Also, these individuals are often hyperflexive.

Sensory Systems

The child with Down syndrome tends to be over- or under-responsive to sensory input.   When she is under-responsive, her awareness of input is diminished so that she is not adequately aroused and focused for learning. When she is over-responsive, she interprets sensory input as unpleasant or uncomfortable and she may avoid those items, activities, or sensations.

The child with Down syndrome may have dysfunction in one or more sensory systems. She may react differently at different times and with different stimuli. She may also have difficulty integrating information and input from the various sensory systems.

Hearing Between 65-80% of individuals with Down syndrome have some form of hearing impairment. The hearing loss usually is conductive in nature, but there also is an increased incidence of sensorineural hearing loss. The majority of individuals have hearing loss in both ears, typically within a mild to moderately severe range. Hearing loss can contribute to lower cognitive and speech-language functioning.

Individuals with Down syndrome are at increased risk for otolaryngologic and audiologic disorders due to congenital malformations and diseases of the nose, sinuses, oral cavity, nasopharynx, larynx, and ears. This population is more likely to develop hearing and otology disorders than other people with mental retardation.

Otolaryngologic concerns may include structural abnormalities, narrow ear canals that can become blocked with cerumen, frequent recurrent otitis media with middle ear fluid accumulation, eustachian tube and tympanic membrane dysfunctions, ossicular abnormalities, and persistent rhinorrhea. Individuals with Down syndrome have upper respiratory, ear, nose and throat infections much more frequently than the general population, although this frequency does decrease with age. This may be secondary to depressed immune function.

Vision Visual problems are fairly common. Twenty to 50% of individuals with Down syndrome have strabismus (i.e., muscle imbalance problems) that causes one or both eyes to turn outward or inward. Nystagmus (i.e., involuntary movements of the eyes) occurs in 10-20% of individuals with Down syndrome. Near- or farsightedness is common and there may be some abnormalities of the cornea. Cataracts develop with advancing age in 40-50% of individuals, although surgical intervention is not necessary in many cases.

Tactile Many people with Down syndrome have difficulty with sensory awareness and tactile feedback. In addition, there may be difficulty processing sensations in the mouth which can contribute to speech difficulties. The individual may be hyposensitive to touch, hypersensitive, or have mixed sensitivity.

Proprio-ceptive Proprioceptive information is that which arises from one's own movements, the sensations generated from muscles and joints. The individual with Down syndrome may be hyporesponsive or hyperresponsive. This creates an altered ability to feel the position of the body or in awareness of body movements and positions, especially in the legs, feet, and face. There may be difficulty with grading of tasks (i.e., controlled increments of movement or positioning). Some may avoid weight-bearing activities.

Vestibular Individuals with Down syndrome tend to use a wide-based gait to give a more secure base of support. There may be decreased balance and protective reactions. There may be gravitational insecurity.

Sensory Integration These individuals tend to have difficulty processing information from more than one channel or sense at a time and then integrating this information. For example, they have marked difficulty with language learning, a skill that involves the ability to simultaneously process and organize input from more than one sense. In essence, they have difficulty learning while simultaneously watching, listening, and doing.

Health Considerations

Otolaryn-gologic concerns
- stenotic (narrow) ear canals that can become blocked with cerumen
- abnormalities of the tympanic membrane
- eustachian tube dysfunction
- ossicular abnormalities
- inner ear abnormalities
- recurrent otitis media with fluid accumulation
- hearing deficits
- mouth breathing due to enlarged adenoids/tonsils or recurrent allergies or colds
- frequent upper respiratory infections

There is a need for frequent hearing screenings in this population, both pure tone and tympanometry. Ear infections, fluid, and excessive ear wax should be treated aggressively to prevent hearing loss, ossicular erosion, and other middle and inner ear problems.

Tonsillectomy reduces tongue protrusion only when the tonsils are truly enlarged and contributing to the problem. Removing the adenoids doesn't help ears, mouth breathing, or throat infections as it does in the typically-developing population because of the small oral cavity, small nasal cavity, and recurrent upper respiratory infections. Children with Down syndrome can be at significant risk for velopharyngeal incompetence following adenoidectomy.

Orthopedic It is common to see subluxation and dislocation of the cervical spine, hips, and knees as well as foot problems. Most orthopedic problems are due to abnormality of the collagen structure and to low muscle tone rather than to congenital abnormalities.

It is important to screen for atlantoaxial instability. Symptoms include head tilt and a limited range of motion in the neck. This condition is often asymptomatic. Pueschel

(1992) recommends radiologic examination of the cervical spine beginning at the age of 2½-3 years, with repeated testing at around 8-9 years. Those with asymptomatic atlantoaxial instability shouldn't participate in any sports activity that could injure the neck.

Dental Concerns Because there is a high incidence of periodontal disease, dental visits should begin early. The child should be seen three to four times per year for preventive care. Children with heart conditions should have a course of antibiotics before dental cleanings or procedures to decrease the chances of heart infection.

Sleep Some individuals may have sleep apnea. There may be a decrease in serotonin levels, which may make it difficult to regulate sleep-awake cycles.

Hematology There may be an increased incidence of hematologic dysfunction or diseases such as low platelet counts or leukemia. There is a 15-20 times higher incidence of leukemia, but it still only affects around 1% of the population with Down syndrome.

Thyroid Dysfunction Screening for thyroid dysfunction may be recommended as these disorders are fairly common in the Down syndrome population.

Growth and Development It is fairly common for the child with Down syndrome to be premature and have a low weight and short length at birth. Growth is usually slower than typically-developing peers, secondary to a deficiency of human growth hormone due to hypothalamic dysfunction.

Head size growth is slow and usually follows height patterns which are shorter than for typically-developing children. Adolescents with Down syndrome reach puberty later than their peers. Adults with Down syndrome usually are below the average height of other adults.

Weight gain often is slower than average, but not as slow as height gains. Weight gain is especially slow in those with heart disease. Conversely, obesity is common and may be apparent as early as two to three years of age. Obesity is related to low tone, reduced activity, and reduced height. An optimal weight can be maintained through an active lifestyle and a monitored diet.

Immune Function There is an increased incidence of immunodeficiencies. Individuals with Down syndrome appear to have low T-cell counts (these may be 40% below normal) and the T-cells that are present may not function normally. This may contribute to the greater occurrence of upper respiratory problems; ear, nose and throat infections; and higher incidence of leukemia. Their immunity may also be influenced by other characteristics (e.g., heart disease, pulmonary hypertension, nutritional problems) that would predispose them to infection.

Immune function may decrease with age. Individuals with Down syndrome may benefit from flu and pneumonia vaccines and vitamin A supplements. In addition, there appears to be an increased prevalence of juvenile rheumatoid arthritis which may be due to genetic or immunological factors.

Chapter 3: Learning and the Child with Down Syndrome

This chapter provides specific information about how the child with Down syndrome learns and why he learns in the manner that he does. This information is beneficial when determining a child's specific learning needs and then programming for those needs. This chapter includes:

- characteristic strengths and weaknesses in learning found in Down syndrome, and how these impact learning
- learning principles
- teaching/therapy techniques and strategies to help maximize the teachers', therapists', and parents' abilities to plan intervention and to maximize the child's learning potential

Our cognitive capabilities are used to organize knowledge and to acquire and integrate new and more complex skills. From the beginning, the child with Down syndrome is compromised by the effect of his syndrome and the interrelationship between his biology and his environment. The child's ability to learn is significantly impaired due to his biological differences including deceleration of:

- the growth of the brain
- the myelinization of the central nervous system
- the growth and effectiveness of synapses and neurotransmitters
- the maturation of the frontal and temporal lobes and cerebellum

When these differences are paired with an environment that may not view the child's ability to learn in a positive manner, the result is that learning is not only a difficult process, but also a different process than that of his typically-developing peers.

The structural and functional deficits and differences in the brain of a child with Down syndrome produce widespread disruption and changes in the way he learns. These differences display themselves in multiple learning and memory system differences and deficits; in different learning patterns, styles, and pathways; and in differences not only in the quantity that the child learns, but also in the quality of what he learns. These brain differences often do not support ordered and stable learning. Instability of learned information is a hallmark characteristic in the learning patterns in children with Down syndrome. These deficits and differences in brain function and the degree of dysfunction varies widely within the Down syndrome population.

Each child with Down syndrome is truly unique and the impact on his general cognitive skills, learning ability, auditory processing skills, communication skills, personal/social skills, behavior, and academic skills can vary greatly from individual to individual. Individuals with Down syndrome may function from the near-normal range to the severely mentally handicapped range, but most fall within the mild to moderate level of mental handicap.

19

Though they learn differently, individuals with Down syndrome are capable of achieving at higher levels than previously thought. It is up to the professional to determine the individual child's strengths and weaknesses, and then use his strengths to enhance learning ability. Implementation of learning principles and strategies appropriate to the individual can make learning more effective and rewarding for the child, family, and professional.

Strengths

The following are often strengths for the individual with Down syndrome.

General Learning

- usually follows the developmental sequence of typically-developing children
- is a fairly efficient learner as an infant
- is able to continue to learn throughout life
- may develop fairly high skills (The syndrome itself does not put a fixed ceiling on ability to learn.)
- achieves higher levels of learning than expected in the past, especially with early intervention

Processing Skills

- demonstrates relatively strong visual processing, including visual motor sequencing and memory skills
- demonstrates relatively good visual and motor decoding skills

Communication Skills

- often demonstrates age-appropriate babbling, imitation, and vocalization skills
- tends to demonstrate good gestural skills
- often demonstrates knowledge of vocabulary and language that is commensurate with his mental age through the first five years
- acquires words using the same "rapid mapping" system as typically-developing children. Once a child with Down syndrome understands approximately 20 words, he is able to figure out what a new word means much the same as his typically-developing peers.

- tends to present strong semantic skills, especially receptively

Personal/Social Skills and Behavior

- demonstrates good skills in the areas of personal and social communication and interaction
- demonstrates fairly good adaptive skills
- demonstrates the same range of personality and behavior attributes as seen in typically-developing peers
- enjoys peer and adult interaction
- has good social skills that decelerate less than his IQ; they remain a strength

Academic Skills

- often learns to read, and tends to demonstrate early sight vocabulary skills
- can learn to write with persistence and practice
- can learn to spell, although spelling ability usually is consistent with the child's ability to read

Weaknesses

When discussing weaknesses in learning of the individual with Down syndrome, it is important to include those learning weaknesses found in the mentally handicapped population in general. Children with mental handicaps generally possess a less reactive central nervous system. Deficits may include:

- poor generalization and consolidation of information, and difficulty with abstract thinking and spontaneous learning
- difficulty with self-regulation, inhibition, planning ability, motivation, pursuance of a specific task, task persistence, as well as poor responsiveness and low initiative
- immature play skills
- deficits in auditory processing skills in the areas of short term memory, sequential memory, figure-ground, and attention
- deficits in the use of abstract language and word-retrieval skills

General Learning

- tends to fall within the mild to moderate range of retardation
- presents global delays in learning, progresses more slowly, and achieves a lower level of development than his typically-developing peers
- has deficits in short term memory
- has significant difficulty maintaining a steady developmental rate of learning
- generally demonstrates low awareness and low reactivity to changes in his environment
- may demonstrate difficulty in maintaining attention and may be easily distracted
- may demonstrate difficulty maintaining and coordinating the ability to attend to the speaker or action, process the information, and respond appropriately
- appears to have reduced activity of the central and peripheral transmission systems, which in part controls how he receives and reacts to stimulation. The child with Down syndrome has a different and less efficient system to work with which makes it difficult to perceive, receive, process, organize, and use information. He finds it difficult to integrate information from different sensory systems, to store information received, and to consolidate new information with previously learned knowledge.
- tends to become a more reluctant learner with age. Even with consistent support, he tends to become a more passive learner, to demonstrate instability in learning, to lose skills already stabilized, and to avoid new learning. Motivational problems are common and often are displayed as learning avoidance and/or failure by default.
- may demonstrate poor task persistence

Impact on General Learning

The strengths and weaknesses presented have direct impact on the individual's ability to learn.

- has inherent difficulties learning new skills. Many of his learning problems are a direct consequence of the effect of the extra chromosome on brain development. A child with Down syndrome experiences more failure and skills take longer to master than the typically-developing child.

- shows relatively normal abilities in learning and memory as an infant, but doesn't possess full learning potential due to differences in brain development and inadequate cerebral specialization. Differences are seen as early as six months of age. Learning gaps occur within the first year.
- is unable to maintain the developmental rate of his typically-developing peers. The individual with Down syndrome demonstrates low arousal and reactivity; passive learning; inconsistent task performance; missed or avoidance of opportunities to learn; difficulties with organization, consolidation and generalization of information; instability of learned skills; poor short term memory; poor problem solving skills; and reduced motivation to learn.
- follows a different pattern of learning than the typically-developing child. He may demonstrate periods of slow progress or no progress, followed by acquisition of new skills. In other children with Down syndrome, cognitive development may be slow, but steady throughout childhood. Many individuals with Down syndrome continue to acquire new skills with continued education and intervention and their mental age continues to increase steadily up to a point. Plateaus in learning in the typically-developing child usually represent a time for consolidation of newly-learned skills. This may not be the case for the child with Down syndrome. During these periods, he may consolidate some new skills, but lose previously learned skills.
- often has an average IQ just below the normal range as an infant. By school age, the IQ level is more likely to be within the mild to moderate range of mental handicap, although some children can present with severe mental handicaps. IQ scores for some children with Down syndrome tend to decline with age.
- tends to fail to make the most of his learning potential and of learning opportunities. Deficits in exploratory behavior, a passive nature, avoidance of learning, failure by default, and failure to demonstrate skills that he has shown previous success with lead to weaknesses in his natural learning ability.
- has difficulty with abstract thinking
- is not a flexible learner. His inability to use different sensory systems simultaneously, paired with slow

reaction time and cognitive deficits, make flexible learning difficult.

- demonstrates low awareness, low persistence to tasks, and distractibility; therefore, it is more difficult for him to master basic skills. This leads to instability of learning and difficulty with effective integration and generalization of new information and skills.

- doesn't demonstrate consistent mastery of skills. Inconsistency may be due to loss of skills, processing deficits, task avoidance, or failure by default. When planning for appropriate intervention, it is often difficult to assess what the child truly knows and doesn't know.

- often presents low task engagement and persistence due to frequent failures, and may use strategies to divert attention from the task being presented. These strategies may include "party trick" behavior (e.g., acting cute), outright task refusal, evasive tactics, or temperament changes.

- demonstrates learned helplessness which can be a result of lower expectations of others and manipulation of others to get them to do for him what he can do for himself

- may avoid tasks that he was successful with or has shown competence with earlier. This may lead to incomplete learning and lack of practice, which affects mastery and consolidation of skills.

- tends to be a more passive learner (e.g., more of a "watcher" than a "doer")

Processing Deficits

- presents significant deficits in processing sensory information when compared to other mentally handicapped individuals and typically-developing children
- tends to process information more slowly
- exhibits difficulty integrating information from various sensory modalities
- presents deficits in the ability to encode and decode sensory information
- exhibits visual processing deficits in the areas of visual monitoring and scanning and matching by size and pattern. Visual perception skills decline with age.
- exhibits auditory processing deficits in the areas of recall of auditory information, auditory reception and

processing (e.g., interpretation and categorization), short and long term auditory memory, and auditory figure-ground. There is a latency in responding to longer, more complex information and decreased auditory comprehension; auditory sequential memory; and auditory verbal skills. Auditory processing skills may be affected by the pattern of repeated ear infections and hearing loss.

- may have difficulty learning the same as a typically-developing child because of auditory processing deficits and the transient nature of language. Auditory information is often presented too rapidly for the child's processing system to accommodate.

- tends to experience tactile processing deficits including distorted sensory awareness to touch and tactile feedback, and difficulty processing sensations in the mouth. These children may demonstrate hypo- or hypersensitivity to touch.

- exhibits proprioceptive processing deficits that may include decreased awareness of the body in space, decreased perception of changes in body positioning, and difficulty with graded movements

- exhibits vestibular processing deficits that may include decreased protective and balance reactions and gravitational insecurity

- exhibits sensory integration deficits that may include difficulty in the ability to perceive, interpret, and organize sensory information from the body and the environment. Sensory integration abilities may be affected by the child's general low awareness and reactivity and his difficulty processing information from more than one sensory system at a time.

Impact of Processing Deficits

Processing deficits can contribute to difficulty mastering basic skills, which is a characteristic of Down syndrome.

- may be slow to orient to auditory stimuli, which causes the child to miss or receive partial information; thus, significantly impacting the child's ability to learn and to develop language
- may miss learning opportunities because they go by too quickly for the child to note, process, and respond. He tends to present lower levels of arousal, reactivity, and latency in processing, which can be responsible for missing or being unaware of many

learning opportunities and changes within his environment.
- is often slower to respond to requests and questions
- has difficulty processing information from more than one sensory system at a time which significantly affects the child's ability to remember, rehearse, consolidate, and generalize information and skills. The simultaneous reception, processing, and integration of information of each sensory system is critical to learning and development.
- may have an ability to learn that is significantly impaired by attention deficit. This interferes with development of the "listen-look-respond" pattern, a foundation skill for learning.
- tends to learn best using the visual channel due to the multiplicity of deficits in processing auditory and other types of information
- demonstrates problems with perception and interpretation of sensory information in the mouth that can interfere with development of skilled oral-motor patterns of movement for feeding and speech

Communication Skills

- presents uneven receptive and expressive language skills, with receptive skills being higher. Particular difficulty is noted in the areas of syntax and morphology, which may be related to deficits in phonological awareness and memory.
- demonstrates difficulty mastering communication commensurate with cognitive skills
- demonstrates deficits in higher-level pragmatic skills
- demonstrates latency in response time
- demonstrates difficulty developing speech skills
- demonstrates difficulty comprehending and using abstract language

Impact on Communication Skills

- presents significant language processing deficits; inefficient organizational skills; difficulty comprehending spatial, quantity, and temporal concepts; and difficulty comprehending complex utterances and abstract language
- demonstrates difficulty in mastering language, both spoken and written forms, although variability exists. Syntax, morphology, and abstract language are particularly difficult.

- tends to demonstrate expressive language deficits. The young child tends to use gestures to communicate rather than words. Other expressive deficits include latency in response, avoidance of responding to questions and requests, difficulty with word retrieval and vocabulary use, use of non-specific words, difficulty with formulation of responses, and difficulty using complex language.
- exhibits pragmatic deficits that include making verbal and nonverbal requests; initiating conversation; topic selection and maintenance; making conversational repairs; taking the listener's knowledge into account; and reading body language, facial expressions, and social cues.
- tends to use concrete vocabulary and talk about the here and now
- exhibits language deficits that can contribute to declines in learning at later ages
- exhibits social development that becomes more dependent on language with age. Language deficits contribute to the decline in social skills seen at later ages.

Personal/Social Skills and Behavior

- has increased risk for developing challenging behaviors if functional communication skills aren't developed
- is more likely to present disruptive behaviors, attention deficit, and oppositional and aggressive behaviors than the typically-developing child
- tends to be less responsive, demonstrates less intensive responses, takes fewer initiatives, and often does not take the lead in social interactions
- demonstrates immature play skills secondary to cognitive, language, and processing deficits

Impact on Personal/Social Skills and Behavior

The diagnosis of Down syndrome can cause parents, educators, siblings, and peers to have low expectations for appropriate social, emotional, and learning skills. Low expectations may lead to reduced achievement, low independence, low self-esteem, and learned helplessness in which the child with Down syndrome tends to have others do for him what he can do for himself.

23

- experiences more difficulty and failure than the typically-developing child when learning basic skills. He also experiences difficulty with maintenance of skills learned. This difficulty learning and maintaining skills may result in the child losing interest in learning, developing reluctance, and actual avoidance of learning. This in turn has a negative impact on his self-esteem, confidence, desire, and motivation to learn.
- may demonstrate avoidance of tasks which may lead to the child developing evasive behaviors or failure by default. He may learn to use these behaviors because it is easier and less painful to fail on purpose than to try and fail.
- may demonstrate less mature play than his same age peers. He tends to look at toys rather than actively play, watch others play rather than engaging in the play, follow another child's lead in play, play alone, miss social cues in play, respond too slowly, and have difficulty creating play schemes.
- may not develop active interaction skills that promote peer relationships because of reduced expectations, a tendency to be a passive observer, and a pattern of avoidance behaviors
- tends to demonstrate immature behaviors rather than developing more age-appropriate ones

Academic Skills

- demonstrates difficulty learning to read and write due to cognitive, motor, and sensory deficits
- demonstrates deficits in auditory processing skills which can make learning to read difficult, particularly when a phonetic approach is used as the sole means of teaching reading
- tends to experience difficulty learning to write because of generalized hypotonicity; loose or lax joints; lack of strength in the hands and fingers; visual problems including visual perception deficits and difficulty with eye-hand coordination; difficulty with motor skills; motor memory planning and control deficits; and difficulty with spatial relationships
- demonstrates difficulty learning math concepts and skills
- exhibits difficulty with higher-level academic skills because of language and cognitive deficits. Higher level academics are very language dependent.

Impact on Academic Skills

The variability in skills makes the educational process a highly individualized one, requiring careful planning, monitoring, and adaptations to meet the child's current and long-term needs.

- achieves at lower academic levels than his peers
- often has difficulty mastering higher-level academic skills because of an acceleration of cognitive, processing, and language requirements beginning in the mid-elementary years
- is usually most successful learning to read using a functional reading approach that establishes an early sight vocabulary. Following the establishment of a core sight vocabulary, the child may then go on to successfully learn to read using a phonetic reading approach.
- tends to lose basic skills and demonstrates difficulty consolidating and generalizing established skills, which results in gaps in knowledge and performance
- may learn to write, but requires more practice than other children. Motor, sensory, and tone issues need to be addressed for the child to be successful.

When identifying and using reinforcers, make sure they are salient. A child with Down syndrome may not view reinforcers in the same way as his peers. The child may not be able to identify the contingencies, may not work for the same type of reinforcement, or be reinforced on the same schedule as the typically-developing child.

Down syndrome has a significant impact on every area of development, but especially on cognitive development and communication skills. The impact of Down syndrome on the child's ability to learn can not be predicted with accuracy. It will vary with the individual child's cognitive skills, degree of sensory impairment, maintenance of optimum health, level of environmental stimulation, and level of appropriate and continued intervention.

The child with Down syndrome has a difficult time establishing basic skills to form a foundation for future learning. He learns more slowly, uses different paths to learning, and may follow a different progression in skill development. Consequently, the educational program must be specifically designed and the environment structured to consistently facilitate learning, prevent loss of previously mastered skills, and assist in consolidation and generalization of skills.

Intervention

The following principles and strategies are presented to facilitate learning in the individual with Down syndrome.

1. **Monitor and maintain health for optimal learning potential.** The individual with Down syndrome has numerous health issues that can affect learning. Monitoring and maintaining health should be a team effort with parents and professionals working with the doctors to insure the best health for learning.

   Strategies include:
   - Periodic Health Screening Schedule: a log of hearing, vision, thyroid, and general health screenings and results
   - Health Monitoring Chart: a chart to record dates and results of screenings, doctor visits (blood work, shots, etc.), growth statistics, and illnesses
   - Health Alert: update current health status with notes to assist professionals working with the child to plan more effectively, to be aware of health changes that may affect performance, and to indicate changes in scheduling or referrals made

2. **All sensory impairments of the child must be identified, assessed as to severity and impact, and addressed for the child to reach his maximum learning potential.** Using the child's areas of strength can provide support for areas of sensory impairment and promote learning.

3. **A team approach is effective in meeting the needs of individuals with Down syndrome.** The team may include parents, caregivers, teachers, therapists, social workers, psychologists, nurses, dietitians, and doctors. The team provides the child with support, guides the intervention process, and coordinates services. Educational plans are reviewed at predetermined periods. Team members can evaluate progress, solve problems, develop strategies, and consult on the planning of future goals and objectives.

4. **It's important to understand the developmental patterns of the typically-developing child when planning intervention for the child with Down syndrome.** Though the child with Down syndrome often learns differently, he may follow a typically-developing sequence of learning. An understanding of traditional developmental milestones serves as a guide to determine where the child is developmentally, to identify specific skill sequences for effective intervention, and to identify the functional skills he will need to effectively interact with his environment and his peers. (See *Milestones for the Typically-Developing Child*, pages 133–148.)

5. **Start early to maintain the child's developmental rate for learning.** Cognitive development tends to slow with age in the child with Down syndrome. Intervention needs to start early to help parents understand their child's areas of strengths and weaknesses, the types of support required for optimal learning, and effective intervention at home.

   Strategies include:
   - building basic skills through practice
   - providing treatment to minimize sensory impairments
   - building attention and response skills
   - providing the child with many learning experiences
   - being positive about the child's learning ability

6. **Therapy should be child-centered to maximize learning.** For optimal learning to occur, the child must share in the selection, direction, and control of the activity. This will promote on-task behavior and attention to the activity.

   Strategies include:
   - keeping tasks relatively short
   - providing activities that are fun, active, and flexible
   - embedding new information into established, predictable routines
   - changing activities frequently during the session
   - frequent review of new skills during functional tasks
   - following the child's lead, using his interests

7. **It's important to have a complete profile of the child's skills before intervention begins.** The profile should include current assessment information, medical and developmental histories, current educational plans and needs, behavior observations and concerns, parent/teacher concerns, specific health problems and needs, learning strengths and weaknesses, and the child's particular interests. This profile can be updated as needed by all members of the team to denote progress or areas of concern.

8. **Determine how the child learns best.** Identify the child's learning style, which includes his learning strengths and weaknesses. Use the child's strengths to support optimum learning.

   Strategies include:
   - using the strength of the visual channel to decrease the transient nature of auditory and tactile information
   - using visual support in the classroom by incorporating pictures and printed words to:
     ▸ organize the classroom (e.g., place pictures on shelves to denote where materials go)
     ▸ denote different work areas
     ▸ signal for help, change in activity, personal needs, or completion of a task
     ▸ make transitions during the day or to move from one activity/location to another
     ▸ make job charts to track jobs completed
     ▸ show a job sequence of each step required in completing a task (page 28)
     ▸ present a work menu to aid in job, task, or activity selection (page 28)
     ▸ list classroom rules
     ▸ make progress charts, progress bulletins, telegrams, brag books, and communication books
   - rehearsing or reviewing a task before or after completion
   - using manual signs and gestures to support weak areas of processing
   - signaling the child of changes in routine or activity by blinking the lights to get attention, using music or a song to signal that it's time to move to the next activity, or using a timer to signal the end of an activity

9. **Intervention should begin at the child's current level and build new skills onto established skills.**

10. **Promote attending skills.**

    Strategies include:
    - using primary reinforcers
    - using verbal and physical prompts (fade with time)
    - reducing distracters
    - using favorite activities
    - beginning with brief tasks
    - changing tasks often
    - incorporating action into tasks
    - slowly increasing attending time and requirements

11. **Structure intervention so the child will be successful by presenting new information in small, attainable steps.**

    Strategies include:
    - analyzing tasks and breaking them into small sequential steps
    - having the child master each step before starting the next
    - providing appropriate feedback and reinforcement
    - using the stronger learning channel to support and cue the weaker channels
    - moving at the child's rate and gradually increasing complexity to facilitate the child's continued cooperation
    - stopping action, looking expectantly, and waiting to cue the child to make a response
    - dropping back to a point where the child is successful if he experiences difficulty
    - starting and ending each session with success

12. **Keep the activity and interaction going.** Avoid turn dominance, dead-end contacts (i.e., asking questions that do not require the individual to respond), mismatch on turn-taking (i.e., taking more turns than the individual), and avoid using a didactic communication style (i.e., a conversational style that doesn't allow the individual to be an equal partner in the activity).

    Strategies include:
    - using balanced turns (i.e., Don't dominate.)
    - pausing and looking expectantly for a response

- cueing for a response
- balancing and matching the level of the individual's communication
- reducing the number of questions asked
- using natural opportunities for learning
- incorporating the techniques of stalling, sabotage, and misunderstanding
- using chaining

13. **Help the child make successful transitions.**

Strategies include:
- using a predictable schedule of activities
- providing visual support by using pictures of activities, areas, or places
- using a picture timeline of the daily schedule
- using a picture or object to cue transition time
- preparing the child for a change by alerting him with a verbal or visual cue a few minutes prior to the change

14. **Intervention goals and objectives must be functional and developmentally appropriate.**

15. **Teach functional daily routines to stimulate consolidation and generalization of skills.** Daily routines provide consistency and predictability as well as a framework for learning and rehearsing skills in functional ways.

16. **Manipulate the environment to maximize learning and the use of skills.** Changes in the familiar and predictable environment can be used as important tools for learning. These changes can effectively be used to teach, model, rehearse new skills, and review established skills.

Strategies include:
- manipulating the environment to elicit a specific response by changing the setting, objects, people, typical sequence, or way of responding. For example:
  - ▶ Have the child set the table, but don't give the child the forks or enough napkins.
  - ▶ When getting dressed, put out only one sock or shoes that don't match.
  - ▶ When brushing teeth, give the child the brush, but no toothpaste.

- ▶ When doing a cutting task, give the child paper, but no scissors.

17. **Make the child's environment conducive to learning and communication by making it language-rich.** Talking about and describing actions, objects, and activities and allowing the child to have hands-on experiences has a positive impact on learning and communication development. As the child ages, he needs to continue to have a variety of experiences and opportunities that stimulate further learning.

18. **Increase and maintain compliant behavior.**

Strategies include:
- using short tasks incorporating engaging activities and manipulatives
- breaking activities into small attainable steps
- providing a visual task schedule (e.g., pictures of tasks attached to a sheet of paper with spaces indicating Job 1, Job 2, etc.; pictures of tasks attached to a clothesline with clothespins) or work folder (page 28)

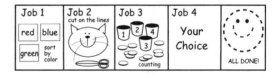

- using total communication for important words like "Stop!, Come here," and "Hot!"
- providing appropriate prompts and cues as needed
- using salient reinforcers and contingencies
- alternating preferred tasks with non-preferred tasks
- using peer models

19. **Foster on-task and task completion behavior.**

Strategies include:
- maintaining a consistent rate of presentation
- keeping the interaction going
- changing tasks frequently
- incorporating action activities
- using fun and interesting activities
- coordinating tasks so each flows meaningfully and naturally into the next

- using humor and a positive, engaging manner
- using the individual's interests as a vehicle to obtain the necessary amount of repetition and drill to learn and stabilize a skill
- incorporating new tasks in established daily tasks or jobs
- providing the child with choices of materials, activities, and activity sequences
- embedding practice into common games like Hide-and-Seek or card games
- including peers and/or siblings in activities
- allowing the child to make choices of tasks, sequences of tasks, and materials used. Make a visual work menu or job bank to facilitate choices.

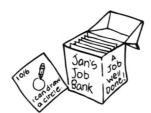

- providing an "All-Done" box for the child to put pictures of completed tasks in
- providing cues within the environment to lead the child to success (e.g., number learning centers so the child follows them chronologically)
- using pictured job sequence strips, folders, or menus

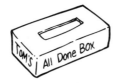

- using a daily activity chart of choices of activities
- using reminder strips, chore charts, or homework charts of things to be done and the order to do them
- using a visual chart so the child has a visual representation of work to come and his progress in completing it
- using task completion charts for motivation (e.g., dot-to-dots, task maps, color in pictures)

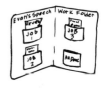

- using work folders (e.g., folders with several pockets and job cards that are placed in an "all done" pocket when completed)
- using a "Hard Worker" chart to show completed tasks with stars or checks
- providing tokens or punches on a timecard for each job completed (Note: Jobs can be worth differing amounts depending on difficulty or length. The jobs that the child does not like can be worth more tokens or the child can do his favorite thing if he completes a task he doesn't like.)

20. **Play is an important vehicle for learning and language development.** Through play, the child explores and learns about his world.

There is a positive relationship between the level of the play skills a child attains and the level of social, language, and cognitive skills that he develops.

The child develops through stages of play the same way as he develops through stages of learning and language development. Therapeutic use of play, where goals and objectives are embedded in the play structure, is an important therapy strategy to use with children.

Strategies include:
- playing at the child's developmental level
- teaching the child how to play using:
  assistance in exploration
  modeling
  imitation
  turn taking
  role playing
- teaching vocabulary through play
- teaching social language related to play
- beginning with a few play items and gradually incorporating more
- using varying levels of prompts and cues
- expanding utterances during play
- using balanced turns (i.e., Don't dominate.)
- matching your play model to or slightly above the child's level of play
- following the child's lead
- demonstrating novel ways to play with/use objects

- taking small steps with lots of support
- eliminating distractions
- teaching peers to draw the child into play
- using realistic props
- teaching the child how to combine items in play

21. **Provide multi-sensory cues to enhance learning.** Children with Down syndrome often need cues from more than one modality for optimum learning.

22. **Provide appropriate cues and prompts to promote learning and communication development.** By providing effective cues, the child with Down syndrome can function more successfully and independently in his environment. A hierarchy of cues and prompts should be identified. Multi-sensory cues are particularly effective with the child with Down syndrome.

Strategies include:
- using the maximum amount of cueing or prompting to elicit the response and then beginning to fade cues
- pairing visual cues with auditory cues
- pairing stronger cues (visual) with weaker modalities (auditory)
- stopping the action, watching, waiting, and expecting a response

Types of cues and prompts include:
- Visual cues: reciprocal gaze, gesture, manual sign, hand cues, pictures, time lines, work folders, picture exchange, pacing boards, or use of color to highlight salient features
- Auditory cues: timers, bells, or buzzers to signal start or finish of a task; verbal cues; finger snaps; or music
- Tactile cues: a touch, physical facilitation, hand-over-hand assistance
- Multi-sensory cues: a combination of cues with emphasis on the visual modality may be the most effective

A hierarchy of cues may include:
- using movement toward the correct response to facilitate its selection
- positioning of the correct response to facilitate its selection

- using redundancy
- exaggerating features, attributes, or presentation
- providing more time to respond
- repeating the questions
- asking related questions
- providing additional information
- providing a multiple choice
- using true-false statements

23. **Use a Total Communication approach with the individual with Down syndrome to promote learning.** Using total communication provides support for the child with specific processing and learning deficits by presenting information using several modalities simultaneously. The child with Down syndrome is often more successful using a Total Communication approach, because his stronger sensory systems are paired with his weaker auditory system to increase his ability to learn. (See Chapter 9, pages 119–125.)

24. **Use appropriate reinforcement.** Identify salient reinforcers for the child with Down syndrome and use the least amount necessary to increase the level of the target response. Using appropriate reinforcement helps the child focus on the task and feel good about his work, his progress, and himself. It is important not to overpower the child with reinforcement, and not to let the reinforcement or the schedule of presentation interfere with the learning or therapy objectives.

Strategies include:
- using a variety of reinforcers, paired with verbal praise
- using 100% reinforcement for the young or resistant child
- using an interval schedule of reinforcement for the older child
- changing the schedule or the reinforcers as needed to maintain effectiveness

25. **Have a predetermined plan to deal with errors.** The child with Down syndrome often is reluctant to make multiple attempts. If he makes a mistake, he may refuse to try again or he may demonstrate failure by default.

Strategies include:
- using tasks that are interesting and functional
- breaking tasks into small achievable steps
- using error-free learning
- immediately dropping back to a place where the child can be successful if he demonstrates difficulty
- structuring tasks to maintain the child's attention, engagement, and success
- improving his feelings of accomplishment by:
  - using progress charts, task charts, and/or work folders
  - using worker awards
  - using brag books (e.g., using stickers or pictures of the child to represent successful task completion)
  - using work tokens/job tickets
- incorporating action into activities to keep the child engaged and energized
- using peer tutors
- playfully negotiating to continue work
- changing how the request is presented
- changing the child's mode of response
- making a desired activity contingent on work completion
- keeping the flow of therapy going

26. **Use the child's social skills as a vehicle for learning.** The child with Down syndrome demonstrates relatively strong social and pragmatic skills. Embedding skills in social contexts can provide the child with a pleasant way to work on tasks he tends to avoid. Use and expand social routines to reduce his passive tendency and to encourage him to become a more active learning partner.

    Strategies include:
    - joint action routines (e.g., brushing teeth, setting the table, making a snack)
    - role playing
    - peer and sibling tutors
    - turn-taking games
    - pretend play

27. **Incorporate peers into the learning process as an effective tool to promote interaction.** The Down syndrome child will often attempt more tasks for his peers and siblings than he will for adults. Peer tutors can have significant positive effect on his approach to learning.

    Strategies include:
    - role playing
    - using job buddies (e.g., one or more peers are assigned to complete a job with the child)
    - using study buddies
    - using play buddies (e.g., the peer demonstrates how to play and encourages the child to participate)
    - using team activities (e.g., the child is made part of a team and is guided through completion of the activity by his peers)

28. **Skills need to be specifically taught to the child with Down syndrome because he finds it difficult to build skills through incidental learning.**

    Strategies include:
    - breaking the task down, teaching step-by-step
    - using hands-on experiences
    - using multiple examples
    - using frequent drill and practice
    - exaggerating the presentation
    - providing necessary prompts and cues
    - modeling skills
    - using salient reinforcement
    - starting with concrete examples with controlled variables

29. **Encourage active participation in the child with Down syndrome.** These children often tend to be "watchers" rather than "doers." They need to be fully engaged in activities and interactions in order to learn from them.

    Strategies include:
    - using prompts and cues including physical prompts or hand-over-hand
    - using progressive approximations
    - stopping, waiting, looking, and expecting a response
    - sabotaging the environment by having missing objects, doing things in the wrong order,

completing a common task incorrectly, or putting things where they do not belong
- stalling
- misunderstanding the child
- chaining

30. **Provide repetitive practice.** The child with Down syndrome needs over-teaching to master new skills and to stabilize old skills. Skills need to be reviewed, practiced, and used regularly to maintain and consolidate learning. Repetition and drill may be incorporated into daily activities.

31. **Present information in a manner that promotes organization, consolidation, and generalization of skills.**

Strategies include:
- using developmentally-appropriate tasks and introducing them in a logical sequence (e.g., teaching winter clothing items in winter when the child can actually experience using and selecting them daily)
- breaking tasks into a sequence of small, attainable steps
- drilling and frequently practicing
- organizing activities in a predictable sequence
- using verbal and physical prompts as needed
- using multi-sensory cues to support learning
- using a "scaffolding" approach where new skills are practiced within the support of established skills
- incorporating environmental changes into practice by changing the object, setting, or person
- practicing target skills in natural settings:
  ‣ joint action routines
  ‣ daily home routines
  ‣ chores or responsibilities
  ‣ classroom routines or structure
  ‣ play scenarios
  ‣ role playing
  ‣ stories, storyboards (i.e., stories illustrated in pictures and placed on a board in order), and scripts (i.e., simple narratives or dialogue about activities that assist the child to organize, to practice skills, to retell, or to act out)

- manipulating the child's environment to promote practice or spontaneous use of the target skill

32. **Prepare the child for learning.** Learning is a whole body process. For optimal learning, the child with Down syndrome needs to be alert and physically ready.

Strategies include:
- monitoring his health
- using gross motor activities to provide maximum alertness and attention
- positioning the child correctly to provide stability and alertness
- establishing a listening/learning set for optimum attention and to promote learning behaviors (e.g., maintaining focus, eye contact, active listening, sitting quietly with hands and feet still, sitting up straight)
- using amplification
- using multi-sensory experiences
- using tactile input
- using taste and food to alert the child

33. **Allow the child with Down syndrome time to respond.** Characteristically the child with Down syndrome demonstrates slower response time. He may need cues or prompts to know that a response is expected of him, to be given additional time to make a response, and assistance in formulating the response.

Strategies include:
- securing attention
- slowing the rate of task presented
- pausing to allow the child time to process and respond (i.e., Wait-Look-Listen)
- using multi-sensory cues to prompt the child to respond
- using a cueing hierarchy

34. **Discourage avoidance of learning and learned helplessness.** If the child often experiences failure, he may develop learned helplessness, a hallmark characteristic in Down syndrome. Because many of these children become more passive with age, it is important to encourage them to do what they can and to complete tasks independently.

Strategies include:
- giving the child time to respond
- not doing things for the child that he is capable of doing himself
- allowing the child to make choices and simple decisions
- accepting how the child does a task
- providing needed prompts and cues
- physically assisting as needed
- using successive approximations to task completion (i.e., chaining)
- using a picture sequence to support independent completion of a task
- giving the child daily responsibilities

35. **Focus on the quality of the learning, not the quantity.** Teaching should focus on the quality of information and skills introduced and learned. Skills taught should be functional, should form building blocks as a foundation for future learning, and should improve the child's ability to function in his environment.

36. **Promote a positive attitude and atmosphere in all interactions with the individual with Down syndrome.** A key element to developing and maintaining a positive learning atmosphere is to establish rapport with the child. You and the child are partners in the learning process.

    Strategies include:
    - using developmentally-appropriate tasks
    - making therapy child-centered
    - providing the child with choices
    - using the child's interests as therapy vehicles
    - keeping tasks short and successful
    - reviewing skills frequently
    - using progress charts, brag books, "Show and Tell"
    - incorporating peers in therapy
    - proceeding at a slower pace, allowing the child time to process and respond
    - providing all the cues necessary for success
    - providing immediate feedback and reinforcement
    - starting and ending with success

37. **Have positive expectations for the learning potential of the individual with Down syndrome.** Often, because of the diagnosis of Down syndrome, parents, teachers, therapists, siblings, and peers have preconceived expectations of what the child will be able to accomplish. Just as we expect the typically-developing child to reach his maximum potential, we should also expect the same for the child with Down syndrome. His education should be planned and promoted carefully. It is important to know the limitations that Down syndrome presents, but not to make the limitations the child's expectations.

    Strategies include:
    - treating the child with Down syndrome first and foremost as a child
    - exposing the child to a normal range of experiences
    - allowing the child to try activities and providing the least amount of assistance for him to be successful
    - letting him attempt what peers and siblings do with proper support and assistance
    - integrating him with typically-developing peers
    - involving the child in activities where he can be fully included and successful (e.g., bowling, Tai Chi, T-ball, dance)

38. **Deal positively with behavior.** Start early by establishing rules and setting expectations for the child's behavior.

    Strategies include:
    - maintaining optimal health
    - determining precipitators of negative behaviors
    - being aware of ways to prevent inappropriate behaviors and how to prevent behaviors from becoming chronic
    - using goals and objectives that are developmentally appropriate
    - simplifying directions, input, and tasks
    - allowing the child to make choices
    - providing the necessary cues for the child to be successful
    - being consistent in implementing behavior rules and consequences
    - redirecting behavior (i.e., calling attention to the positive aspects of behavior rather than the negative by saying things like, "I like the way you

picked up your truck. Now pick up your other toys.")
- using natural consequences or physically assisting the child through the task step-by-step
- reinforcing only those behaviors that you want to be repeated; ignoring others
- immediately dealing with negative behaviors
- selecting salient reinforcement and providing an appropriate schedule
- using time-out
- teaching use of a target behavior in one setting and expanding to others

39. **Maintain active learning throughout life.** Although the rate of learning slows down with increased age, the individual with Down syndrome can and should continue to learn throughout life.

Strategies include:
- maintaining an enriching environment
- keeping the individual active, interested, and exploring the world around him
- helping the individual have goals and interests, continue to develop them, and enjoy life
- giving the individual responsibilities and chores
- helping the individual find a job, when possible
- helping the individual establish peer relationships and join social groups
- helping the individual develop hobbies and leisure time interests such as sports, collecting, group activities, and arts and crafts
- helping the individual join groups (e.g., Special Olympics, Riding for the Handicapped, bowling, dance)

40. **Facilitate early literacy and reading skills.** The use of print with the child with Down syndrome can facilitate his auditory and memory skills, language comprehension, speech skills, and general learning. The child with Down syndrome typically has relatively strong visual and receptive language skills and can develop an early sight vocabulary. Early literacy can be used to support development of communication skills. Some children with Down syndrome can begin to read sight words as early as two-three years of age.

Strategies include:
- selecting highly salient, functional words as early sight words; starting early to teach first sight words
- pairing pictures and print to create:
  - ▸ albums of family names and acquaintances
  - ▸ theme books
    - My First Words
    - Things I like
    - Places I Go
    - Things I Can Do
    - School Words
  - ▸ classroom dictionary
  - ▸ flash cards
  - ▸ card games
  - ▸ word banks
- using match, select, sort, and label techniques to teach reading
- using a language experience approach by creating simple stories about daily routines, activities, or interests using pictures and print
- selecting a special word for the day
- using print paired with pictures throughout the child's environment by labeling objects and places
- using functional reading tasks (e.g., survival signs, newspaper ads, shopping lists, labels, menu planning, recipes)
- using toys and games that use pictures and print (e.g., Lotto, Bingo)
- using words and pictures to provide visual steps to complete a task
- helping the child build phrases and sentences to read with sight words he knows
- introducing the alphabet and letter sounds if the child has successfully established a sight vocabulary (i.e., start with the first letters of the child's name and established sight words)
- making alphabet books (e.g., words that start with the letter A)
- making flash cards for letter recognition
- making books and reading a daily activity
- using all necessary cues and prompts to make the child successful
- providing a means to practice and rehearse what the child is unable to generate on his own
- using print rather than traditional models and pictures (may be more productive to teach some skills with print)

41. **Foster writing skills.** The child with Down syndrome can learn to write, but often experiences more difficulty than his typically-developing peers. He may require adapted teaching strategies.

Strategies include:
- encouraging the child and praising all efforts
- waiting for the child to show interest before teaching pre-writing skills
- positioning the body correctly for stability and mobility
- fostering appropriate grasp of writing materials
- providing hand-over-hand assistance as needed
- providing experience with developmentally appropriate crayons, paint, markers, pencils, and pens
- drawing pictures together
- progressing slowly in fun, functional tasks
- incorporating drawing and writing in age-appropriate art and craft activities
- using developmentally-appropriate tracing and copying activities
- using successive approximations
- making writing and drawing fun, functional, and meaningful with tasks like:
  ‣ the child's name
  ‣ simple thank-you notes or gift cards
  ‣ holiday cards
  ‣ grocery and shopping lists
  ‣ party invitations
  ‣ writing notes for siblings
  ‣ taking orders for snacks
- using a computer and/or typewriter for children who experience difficulty learning to write

42. **Foster math skills.**

Strategies include:
- using manipulatives to make math functional and concrete
- using hands-on math experiences such as giving each child at the table a napkin at snack time
- using daily tasks to practice math skills
  ‣ cooking
  ‣ shopping at the grocery
  ‣ setting the table
- introducing math skills in developmental sequence
  ‣ introducing early quantity concepts (e.g., *one, all, none, all gone*)
  ‣ introducing rote counting
  ‣ using one-to-one correspondence
  ‣ counting objects
  ‣ introducing number concepts
  ‣ matching sets
  ‣ recognizing numbers
  ‣ ordering numbers
  ‣ introducing later-developing quantity concepts (e.g., *more, less, many, several, each*)

Chapter 4: Feeding and Oral-Motor Skill Development

Many sensory and motor skills are involved in the development of efficient and mature feeding skills. Feeding and oral-motor skills are interrelated. A deficit in one area can affect the development in another.

Children develop a variety of feeding skills over time. Each skill is practiced until it can be performed automatically with efficiency and is integrated with other established skills. For a child to be a successful eater, the following components are necessary:

- normal sensory processing skills (registration, reactivity, integration, and modulation)
- postural stability through the trunk, shoulder girdle, head, and neck
- coordinated suck-swallow-breath pattern during feeding
- synchrony of the jaw, lip, cheek, and tongue functions to move liquid and food from the front of the mouth back to the pharyngeal area for swallowing
- coordinated swallow pattern
- appropriate strength, stability, and movement of the oral structures
  - ‣ jaw strength, control, stability, and grading
  - ‣ cheek strength
  - ‣ lip control, strength, and seal around breast, bottle, or utensil
  - ‣ tongue control, strength, protrusion, retraction, lateralization, elevation, spread, and groove
- separation of movement (independent tongue movement separate from jaw movement)
- development of appropriate munch, bite, and rotary chew for food grinding and manipulation
- shared synchrony throughout the systems of the body during feeding
- rhythmicity between the caregiver and child during feeding
- reaching, grasping, and releasing for finger feeding and bringing food to the mouth

A feeding disorder can occur when there is a weakness or delay in the development in one or more parts of the system, or in the synchrony between the systems. This can adversely affect oral-motor, feeding, and possibly speech skills. In the Down syndrome population, common contributors to feeding problems or disorders may include the following:

1. global developmental delays

2. poor physical base for feeding
   - hypotonicity
   - poor postural strength; tone; and control of the trunk, head, and neck
   - poor stability and control through the trunk, shoulder girdle, head, and neck
   - weak abdominal muscles affecting trunk stability and respiration
   - poor muscle strength and coordination
   - joint laxity
   - small oral cavity and a high vaulted palate
   - a thick bunched tongue

3. health problems
   - chronic respiratory infections
   - chronic ear infections and otitis media
   - poor nasal breathing
   - enlarged tonsils and adenoids
   - thyroid problems
   - digestive problems
   - constipation

4. sensory and sensory processing deficits
   - hearing
   - vision
   - poor attention, vigilance, and registration (i.e., how the body reacts to different stimuli)
   - low awareness and responsiveness
   - hypo- or hyper-oral sensitivities
   - poor sensory processing (auditory, proprioceptive, and tactile)

5. oral-motor deficits
   - poor integration of the suck-swallow-breath pattern, which can lead to aspiration
   - habitual open mouth posture
   - poor jaw stability, control, grading, and strength for biting and chewing
   - hypotonicity in the lips, tongue, and cheeks
   - delay in developing efficient tongue movement
   - forward tongue carriage or tongue thrust
   - poor tongue tip elevation during food movement and swallowing
   - poor tongue grooving
   - poor tongue lateralization for food movement
   - inefficient cheek, lip, tongue, and jaw coordination
   - poor motor planning
   - poor awareness and efficiency for clearing food from the mouth
   - difficulty with separation of function and movement

6. specific feeding difficulties
   - initial difficulty with suckle/suck
   - initial difficulty establishing feeding rhythm between systems as well as between the child and caregiver
   - difficulty managing solids when first introduced
   - slow to develop chewing; maintains an immature chew longer than their peers
   - tends to reject different food textures
   - tends to overstuff the mouth
   - tends to swallow food before chewing completely
   - tends to not evacuate food well from the oral cavity
   - tends to wash food down with liquid before it is fully chewed

Intervention

The development of feeding skills is a sequential process that gradually develops during the first two years. Some children with Down syndrome will follow the same developmental patterns as their peers, while others will demonstrate delays due to hypotonicity, oral sensitivity, poor oral-motor skills, and anatomical differences.

Knowledge of the general development stages and sequences is important before beginning a feeding program. It is important for parents to know these stages so they can identify when their child is experiencing difficulty and help meet her feeding needs. Parents need information about:

- feeding characteristics of the infant and child with Down syndrome
- how to establish feeding rapport and rhythm to support the child's skills
- how to establish a positive feeding environment
- what, when, and how much to feed
- appropriate positioning for feeding
- effective food presentation methods
- the interrelationship between feeding, oral-motor, and speech skills
- adaptive equipment for feeding (e.g., positioning, seating, utensils)
- how to introduce new foods, including tastes, textures, and temperatures
- specific information about the child's feeding strengths and weaknesses, and feeding goals and objectives

It is important to use a team approach when addressing feeding problems. Working closely with an occupational therapist (OT) and a physical therapist (PT) is important, especially if you have not been trained in feeding and oral-motor facilitation or don't feel comfortable or knowledgeable about the techniques presented.

Feeding Evaluation

Before beginning a feeding program, the child's feeding skills should be assessed using both formal tools and informal observation. A team approach is beneficial having all therapists and the parents working together to identify the child's feeding strengths and weaknesses. The following information should be obtained during the feeding evaluation.

1. A complete background and medical history, including the presence of food and latex allergies.

2. A parent interview to document concerns and feeding problems. Information obtained should include presence or history of choking, coughing, regurgitating while eating; difficulty digesting foods; types of foods the child eats or refuses; the child's efficiency as an eater; the amount of support needed during feeding; positioning during feeding; the feeding schedule; the amount of food taken in; the time it takes to feed the child; the utensils used; and examples of daily menus (to assess the nutritional value of the foods consumed).

3. A feeding observation that should be completed while the caregiver feeds the child. Information obtained should include the interaction between the parent and child; types of food fed and their appropriateness; food presentation strategies used and their effectiveness; utensils used; typical position(s) used during feeding; how the child accepts and manages different liquids, food textures, tastes, and temperatures; and any negative reactions during feeding.

4. A feeding assessment to identify specific feeding problems and the strategies to address them. Areas to assess should include:

   a. examination of the oral mechanism and oral-motor skills for structural and functional abnormalities or differences that could affect feeding and speech
   b. examination of the gag reflex for normal function
   c. effectiveness and synchrony of the stages of swallowing
   d. respiration before, during, and after feeding
   e. identification of oral-motor problems, oral sensitivities, or tactile defensiveness on the face, around the mouth, or in the mouth
   f. trunk, shoulder girdle, and head and neck stability during feeding
   g. synchronicity and efficiency of feeding
      - effectiveness of the bite and chew
      - taking appropriate-sized bites
      - appropriate amount of food in the mouth
      - chewing food completely before swallowing
      - effective use of the lips and cheeks
      - lips closed during chewing
      - effective tongue function for food management and movement
      - efficiency of clearing the oral cavity of food
      - inappropriate use of liquid to wash down food
      - presence of choking, gagging, regurgitation of food or liquid
      - loss of food or liquid through the nose
   h. acceptance and management of various foods, liquids, textures, tastes, and temperatures
   i. the effect of different positions on feeding efficiency (e.g., being held on the parent's lap with the back and head supported or leaning on the parent's arm with chin slightly tucked vs. being seated properly [90-90-90] in an appropriately-sized chair)
   j. the effect of different food presentations (e.g., tapping the child's lips with a spoon and waiting for the child to open her mouth and accept the spoon vs. bringing the spoon straight toward the child and stopping in front of her face, waiting for her to signal that she is ready for another bite)
   k. effective use of feeding utensils, bottle, cup, and straw
   l. awareness of food on the child's lips and in or around the child's mouth
   m. use of arm and hand movements for finger feeding and use of eating utensils

5. A feeding plan to assist the parent and child, and to coordinate the team to meet the child's feeding needs. The plan should follow normal feeding development guidelines, but be specific to meet the individual child's needs. It should document each therapist's role, the child's specific feeding goals and

objectives, a time frame for implementation, and any referrals to be made for medical diagnoses or management.

6. Referrals for specific medical diagnoses or management. If any structural or functional abnormality is found or suspected during the feeding evaluation, appropriate referrals should be made. Referrals should be made to diagnose swallowing deficits (i.e., dysphagia); palatal, pharyngeal, and esophageal structural and functional abnormalities; and gastroesophageal reflux. If there is presence of frequent coughing, nasal loss of liquid, choking, regurgitation, or discomfort after feeding, a referral should also be made.

Feeding Principles, Strategies, and Techniques

It is important to use a team approach when identifying and remediating feeding deficits and to educate parents about their child's special needs. Working with a pediatric OT and PT can maximize skills, time, and efficiency in treatment.

I. **Normalize sensory awareness, reactivity, processing, and response.** Children with Down syndrome typically demonstrate decreased alertness and awareness, decreased oral awareness and processing, oral sensitivity issues, and poor oral-motor skills. For them to be effective eaters, they need to have their bodies and their mouths prepared for feeding.

Because of the child's sensorimotor deficits, she needs to be prepared for eating by increasing her alertness and awareness. The facilitation activities that follow serve to help the child focus her attention and organize her system for eating. Be sure to do all stimulation symmetrically. Once the child is ready, proceed with feeding. Strategies and techniques to prepare the child for feeding include the following:

- To energize the infant, gently bounce her on your knee or lap and/or rock, tickle, or wash the child's face with cool water. The older child can be energized by completing gross motor activities such as running, hopping, jumping,

and dancing. Fast, unexpected, arrhythmic movements can also be alerting.

- To prepare the infant's face, use gentle face pats, taps, or strokes, or massage the cheeks using the hands, a washcloth, or different textures and temperatures. For the older child, use face pats, taps, smacking the lips, blowing kisses, licking the lips, tongue clicks, moving the tongue left to right, and blowing whistles.
- To prepare the infant's oral cavity, allow the infant to chew or suck on her fingers or massage her lips and gums with a finger or washcloth. For the older child, use swabbing; stroking; massaging; or tapping the gums, tongue, and buccal cavities.

Some children demonstrate sensory variations in their oral cavities. Children who present hypo-sensitivity in the oral cavity often demonstrate the following during eating:

- stuffing their mouths
- inefficient chewing and movement of food in the mouth
- not chewing food completely before swallowing
- poor awareness of food left in or around the mouth during eating
- washing food down with liquid
- messy eating

Strategies to normalize sensitivity in the hypo-sensitive child may include the following:

- raising awareness and oral sensation by preparing the child's body, face, and oral cavity before eating
- using tapping, stroking, and swabbing of the lips, gums, tongue, and buccal cavity
- using rapid, irregular stimulation

Children who present hyper-sensitivity in the oral cavity often demonstrate the following problems:

- tactile defensiveness around the face and in the oral cavity

- refusal of face washing
- ticklishness in the oral cavity
- rejection of texture and temperature variations
- can be picky or messy eaters

Strategies to normalize sensitivity in the hyper-sensitive child may include the following:

- use of the infant's or child's hands, fingers, and toys to stimulate the mouth and oral cavity
- determining which type of touch pressure the child prefers. Most prefer deep pressure or firm touch, but some children prefer light touch.
- starting touch experiences at the extremities, then slowly proceeding to the face and mouth. Deep pressure or firm touch is recommended, but assess the child's preference first.
- using your hand or a washcloth to stroke, pat, or tap the face and lips
- once the child accepts stimulation to the face, move to the mouth and inside to the oral cavity
- stroke, massage, and swab the lips, gums, tongue, and buccal cavities
- always explain what you are going to do before and as you do it

For the older child, let her practice on you or a doll before beginning direct stimulation to her face and oral cavity.

2. **Normalize the child's body tone before beginning feeding.** The child with Down syndrome typically demonstrates low tone. Strategies and techniques to increase and normalize tone may include the following:

- completion of gross motor, weight-bearing, and "heavy work" activities such as running, jumping, stretching, dancing, pushing a wagon, or carrying a box of books
- oral-motor activities such as tapping on the face, jaw, lips, and tongue
- rapid manual vibration to the face and lips
- positioning the child correctly

3. **The child with Down syndrome must be positioned for maximum stability through the trunk, shoulder girdle, head, and neck for feeding and eating.**

The young infant should be held in a supine position at approximately a 45-degree angle for bottle-feeding. Her back and trunk should be straight and supported, with the hips bent and flexed, shoulders and arms forward, and the chin tucked slightly. The child's ears should always be above her mouth to safeguard against liquids entering the eustachian tubes and middle ear.

Once the infant develops a strong suck, she should be fed in a more upright position with her head in mid-line and her chin tucked slightly. Bottle-feeding in this position requires the child to suck more strongly and helps to develop stronger lip, tongue, cheek, and jaw function.

When positioning the child for spoon-feeding, self-feeding, or cup drinking, she should be in an upright position with her head in mid-line, her chin tucked slightly, and with a 90-degree angle at the hips, knees, and ankles. Her feet should always be supported. Use of a tray or table allows the child to stabilize her body for feeding.

4. **Children with Down syndrome need assistance in developing a strong suck-swallow pattern.** A normal suck pattern has two stages: suckling and sucking. They should be strong, rhythmical, and efficient. The child must be able to initiate and sustain sucking. Infants with Down syndrome typically present a weakness in this area. They need to develop stronger lip, cheek, tongue, and jaw function and strength, as well as organization and coordination of the feeding mechanism. Ways to facilitate a stronger suck may include:

- selecting an appropriate length, shape, and size of the nipple for bottle-feeding. The hole in the nipple can be modified. It may be best to start with a medium-sized hole in the nipple. As the child develops a stronger suck, the size of the nipple hole should be gradually reduced.

- using a bottle with a liner. This allows the caregiver to squeeze gently to provide assistance in drawing the liquid up into the child's mouth.
- positioning the bottle so that gravity plays a part in the suck, then gradually positioning the bottle so that the child must use a stronger suck
- introducing thickened liquids
- positioning the child in a more erect 90-90-90 position as he gets older
- reducing tongue thrust during sucking by tapping on the center and front of the tongue prior to eating
- teaching straw drinking

  a. Place a straw into the child's favorite drink and put your finger on the top end. This will cause suction and will hold liquid in the straw. Place the straw into the child's mouth and slowly let the liquid drip onto the child's tongue by briefly removing your finger. Continue until the child begins to suck the liquid from the straw.

  As the child develops the ability to suck, gradually lower the angle of the straw until it is in a normal drinking position (i.e., tilt the straw so the end with your finger ends up in the liquid).

  b. Use of a squeeze bottle can assist the child in developing straw drinking. The caregiver can assist the child drawing liquid up into the straw and the child's mouth by gently squeezing the bottle. Assistance can be faded as the child demonstrates an improved suck.

  c. Expand to more challenging straw drinking to facilitate use of a stronger suck. This includes use of commercial juice boxes, thin straws, curly straws, and thicker liquids.

5. **Make sure the environment is conducive to feeding.** Strategies and techniques to establish a conducive environment include the following:

   - correctly positioning the child in a comfortable, stable manner

- preparing the child's body and oral mechanism for feeding
- reducing sensory input and distractions and making sure the environment is familiar, calm, quiet, and supportive for the child so she can focus her attention on feeding. This could include lowering the lights, finding a quiet area, and/or wearing soft textures and muted colors when feeding.
- making feeding and eating an enjoyable, pleasurable, shared experience by developing an ongoing communication with the child during feeding; establishing consistent feeding schedules, sequences, or routines; including the child with the family at mealtime; serving foods that are similar to the rest of the family; and/or using calming music

6. **Help the child develop rhythmicity during feeding.** Children with Down syndrome initially present difficulty establishing a rhythm during feeding. Strategies and techniques include the following:

   - taking time with the child, allowing her to practice and establish this rhythm
   - preparing the child for feeding
   - establishing a feeding routine
   - positioning the child for stability during feeding
   - being sensitive to the child's needs and signals
   - eliminating distracters
   - not rushing feeding (e.g., Allow the child to indicate that she is ready for more before another bite or drink is offered; allow the child time to swallow or chew and swallow a bite before another is offered.)
   - watching for signs and stopping before the child becomes upset. Infants with Down syndrome typically tire easily when eating.

7. **Proper food presentation is important when feeding the child with Down syndrome.** Food presentation strategies include the following:

   - foods presented should be developmentally appropriate for the child's stage of feeding

- presenting food at a temperature that the child accepts
- presenting small spoonfuls, allowing the child time to process them
- presenting food straight on at eye level, not from the side
- using developmentally-appropriate feeding utensils, bottles, and cups
- introducing one new texture or taste at a time
- introducing new tastes and textures gradually by intermixing them with established tastes and favorite foods
- presenting food that is appealing to look at and smells good

8. **Gradually introduce changes in taste, temperature, and texture.** (Note: Children with Down syndrome will take longer to progress from baby food to table food.) Strategies may include the following:

   a. Introduce textures systematically when the child demonstrates the oral-motor skills to manage them (e.g., munching, chewing).

      - Introduce one texture at a time; disperse spoonfuls of new texture between other accepted foods (i.e., alternate spoonfuls of accepted foods with the new texture).
      - Do not try to feed new textures all at once or before feeding an accepted food.
      - Textures can be introduced by thickening liquids with yogurt, applesauce, infant cereals, mashed potatoes, nectar juices, or commercial thickeners.
      - Allow the child to explore textured foods with her hands when introducing new textures.

   b. Introduce textures as early as possible. Sequence of presentation follows:

      - Introduce thickened liquids and pureed foods.
      - When the child demonstrates the ability to munch, introduce mashed vegetables, fruits, and meats.
      - Introduce pureed vegetables, fruits, and meats that contain lumps.

- Introduce chopped or bite-sized foods such as vegetables, fruits, crackers, Cheerios®, and meats, including hamburger.
- Introduce cut-up table foods.

   c. Introduce new tastes.

      - Begin with bland tastes, but take the child's food preferences into account.
      - Mix new tastes with old and gradually fade the old taste.
      - Introduce one new taste at a time.
      - Introduce new tastes when the child is hungry.
      - Gradually introduce a variety of tastes.

   d. Introduce different temperatures.

      - Initially present established or favorite foods at room temperature.
      - Gradually introduce different temperatures to the extremities and the face before offering different temperatures in foods. Probe to see if the child tolerates cool or warm and start there.
      - Let the child explore the food with her hands first before trying to feed it to her.
      - Gradually introduce temperature changes using favorite foods.

9. **Use appropriate eating utensils and techniques to assist the child in developing spoon/fork feeding and cup drinking.**

   a. To facilitate spoon feeding:

      - correctly position the child for eating
      - present the spoon straight on and tap or touch the lip to cue the child to come forward and open the mouth to accept the spoon
      - provide external manual support as needed (i.e., hands and fingers on jaw and face, or use firm pressure under the chin to keep the base of the tongue from moving forward – Morris, 1987)
      - place the spoon straight into the child's mouth and press down lightly on the tongue (vibrating the spoon may reduce a tongue thrust pattern)

- encourage the child to use her upper lip to scrape the food off the spoon by waiting a few seconds for the child to respond once the spoon is in her mouth. Use a physical prompt as needed to get the child to move the upper lip down. Avoid scraping the food off with the child's teeth.
- encourage appropriate tongue placement by tapping on the center and front of the tongue and giving a verbal cue
- use developmentally-appropriate spoons and small spoonfuls
- allow the child time to process the food before offering more
- have older children signal before offering another spoonful

b. To facilitate independent self-spoon feeding:

- initially present foods that will stick to the spoon, making it easier for the child to manage (e.g., mashed potatoes, pudding)
- use adaptive spoons as needed
- break the task down into manageable components, gradually building components and complexity
- use hand-over-hand assistance and gradually fade assistance as the child becomes more proficient
- use dishes with lips or raised edges
- use mats under dishes to keep them in place while the child attempts to fill her spoon

c. To facilitate cup drinking:

- use developmentally appropriate liquids
- use liquids the child likes
- select cups that are the appropriate size for the child and support oral-motor function
- use adaptive cups as needed
- correctly position the child for feeding
- bring the cup to the child's lips, pressing in on the lower lip with the cup
- pour in a small amount of thickened liquid as the child sucks
- encourage retention of the cup with the lips or teeth; tongue should be retracted, not under

the cup. Tap on the center and front of the tongue to encourage retraction.
- encourage the child's use of a lip seal around the cup
- encourage the child to hold the cup; assist as needed
- gradually reduce assistance until the child holds and drinks unassisted

Feeding utensils used to teach and support spoon and cup drinking	
• coated spoons • adaptive spoons • cups with spouts • cut-out cups • cups that control liquid flow • non-spill cups • cups with or without handles • raised edge cups and dishes • weighted cups and dishes	• dishes with suction bottoms • dishes divided into sections • non-skid materials to keep dishes in place during eating • cups and dishes that come in interesting shapes and colors or with pictures or cartoon characters

10. **Keep feeding problems from becoming habitual.**
This can be done by:

- establishing a consistent feeding schedule
- establishing a consistent feeding routine
- establishing mealtime rules as the child gets older
- providing regularly scheduled snacks. Snack time is good for working on making choices and will get the child to the next meal if she has refused an earlier one.
- not rushing the child
- not forcing the child to eat and not getting into power struggles. This sets up behavior problems that can affect the way the child eats throughout her life.

Stay calm throughout feeding. If you become upset or excited, it can reinforce the child's negative behaviors and can promote habitual feeding problems.

Be consistent if the child refuses a food. If the child refuses to eat a specific food or spits it out, don't get upset. Try to determine why. Look at the texture, taste, and temperature of the food(s) being offered. Wait a short time and again present a small spoonful to the child. If the child refuses, wait a few minutes and try again. Try mixing the refused food with a favorite food. Keep portions small. If the child continues to refuse, try again at a later time.

For children with feeding problems, keep a feeding diary to help identify the bases for problems and to document and monitor solutions and progress.

II. **Facilitate oral-motor skills needed for mature and independent feeding.** (For more information on direct oral-motor techniques, see Chapter 8, Appendix A, pages 106–114.)

a. To facilitate biting and chewing along with jaw stability and grading:

- position the child for maximum stability
- prepare the child for feeding
- provide the child with toys of various textures to mouth
- provide external manual support to the jaw by placing the middle finger under the chin, the index finger on the chin below the bottom lip, and the thumb on the side of the face. This support can gradually be faded as the child demonstrates improvement.
- teach biting by placing a thin cracker between the child's front teeth and manually closing the jaw on the cracker so the child bites through it
- facilitate biting and jaw stability by placing a washcloth or food between the child's teeth and have her bite down on it as you gently tug. The cloth can be placed between the front teeth and/or between the molars. Placement can be alternated.
- develop munching by allowing the child to mouth and munch on finger foods and teething toys
- facilitate chewing by placing foods on alternating sides of the mouth in the molar region using manual support as needed
- teach the child to chew thoroughly before swallowing food

- teach the child to take appropriate-sized bites
- introduce a "Snack Cap" to stimulate awareness and active chewing. (It is made of a baseball cap and piece of wide elastic attached to fit snugly, but not tightly, under the child's chin. It is used to provide proprioceptive input and feedback and increases jaw stability during feeding. [Morris, 1987].)

b. To facilitate lip tone and function during eating:

- apply manual vibration along the facial muscles, down to and around the child's lips
- use quick pats, strokes, taps, or stretches to the cheeks and lips
- use sustained blowing activities
- have the child hold an object flat between her lips (not teeth) such as a tongue blade or straw
- have the child suck through straws of different lengths and diameters
- use resistive sucking including milkshakes, semi-frozen drinks, curly straws, or looped aquarium tubing
- encourage lip closure during chewing and drinking using physical prompts or a mirror as needed

c. To facilitate tongue function during eating:

- to raise awareness and sensation, use quick taps or strokes on the tongue right before eating
- to facilitate retraction, tap or use quick strokes on the front and center of the tongue or use a quick forward stretch of the tongue
- to facilitate tongue tip elevation, place food on the alveolar ridge or upper lip and have the child lick it off; also push down on the tip of the tongue and have the child follow the finger up as it is lifted
- to facilitate tongue lateralization, put food between the molars or in the buccal cavities and have the child move it or clear it; also press in on the sides of the tongue and have the child push back for resistance

- to facilitate a tongue groove, stroke and tap the center of the tongue in the middle and come forward to the tip
- to facilitate a tongue bowl, press down on the center of the tongue with a spoon and hold
- to increase tongue strength, see Chapter 8, Appendix A, pages 110–113 for facilitation techniques

d. To facilitate cheek function during eating:

- use quick taps or strokes to the cheeks
- massage the cheeks
- apply tactile stimulation inside the buccal cavities (e.g., swabbing)
- place food in the buccal cavity or between the molars
- lightly squeeze the cheeks to help the child be aware of and to monitor for food stored in the buccal cavity

e. To reduce drooling:

- assess the child's ability to breathe through her nose; check for enlarged tonsils and adenoids
- identify the activities where drooling occurs
- position the child with the back straight and head in mid-line with the chin tucked
- teach the child what *wet* and *dry* mean and how they feel
- increase the child's tone throughout the body and face, including the lips
- apply manual vibration along the course of the facial muscles to the lips and around the lips
- tap the child's lips and jaw line
- use oral-motor techniques that encourage lip closure (e.g., V pressure, lip stroking, mustache press) (See Chapter 8, Appendix A, pages 108–109 for descriptions.)
- use techniques to encourage lip strength such as placing a flat object between the child's lips and holding it, then gently trying to pull it out
- facilitate jaw control, strength, and closure by using jaw resistance activities, biting crackers and celery sticks, biting and tugging, and manually supporting the jaw during feeding

- give the child verbal or visual prompts to close her mouth and swallow
- be positive and reward the child with praise for having a dry mouth
- press a cloth over the wet area and tell the child that her mouth is wet
- use a mirror which allows the child to visually monitor her mouth and wipe it when it is wet
- reduce sugar intake
- use peer models

12. **For the independent eater, teach appropriate, socially-acceptable eating skills.** These skills are very important for the child to be accepted by peers and within the community. Skills to teach include the following:

- wiping own mouth as needed
- taking appropriate-sized bites
- having the appropriate amount of food in her mouth
- chewing with the lips closed
- chewing completely before swallowing
- clearing her oral cavity and mouth of food
- correctly using eating utensils
- using good manners at the table

Ways to teach these skills may include consistent practice and use of skills at home and school during meals, using visual and verbal prompts, and providing a mirror so the child can monitor herself. It may also help to involve siblings and peers as models and/or role-play social scenarios.

> *In general, children with Down syndrome take longer to eat during meals than their typically-developing peers.*

Chapter 5: Motor and Sensorimotor Skill Development

An individual's gross and fine motor skills and sensorimotor skills are important for exploring the world and learning about it. They are also important for development of communication skills. Gross motor skills are important for large movements and locomotion; fine motor skills are important for play skills, object manipulation, self-help, self-feeding, speech, and augmentative communication.

Delay in obtaining motor milestones may contribute to delays in cognitive and language skills in the child with Down syndrome. These children have difficulties with sensorimotor and motor skills secondary to brain differences, neurological deficits, laxity of joints, decreased muscle tone and strength, poor sensory processing, and poor motor planning.

Decreased muscle tone and strength throughout the body contributes to a delay in development of gross and fine motor skills and in oral-motor development. Decreased muscle tone and strength can contribute to the child's tendency to be a watcher rather than a doer. He may be using a great deal of energy just to remain upright against gravity. He may tire out more quickly than other children and may have difficulty sustaining attention. Hypotonia may also contribute to latency of response and a dampening of emotional reactions which impede verbal and nonverbal turn-taking.

Individuals with Down syndrome tend to exhibit joint laxity, excessive hip abduction and external rotation, shoulder girdle instability, asymmetrical or excessive range of motion of movements, and difficulty initiating movement. They tend to avoid weight bearing, weight shifts, and trunk rotation. They also tend to have difficulty with equilibrium, balance, protective responses (e.g., the ability to catch yourself as you fall), and graded muscle movements. All of these factors contribute to the use of a wide base of support in sitting and standing and a delay in locomotion. Most children with Down syndrome walk independently between the ages of 2½-3 years.

Individuals with Down syndrome have difficulty with the planning aspect of motor performance. Their motor-planning ability is affected by their tendency toward hearing loss/fluid and visual problems. It is also affected by slow reaction time, postural and gravitational insecurity, and poor awareness of where their bodies are in space. They also have difficulty processing and integrating sensory information.

Intervention

It is important to develop strength and stability through the trunk in order to facilitate appropriate respiration/phonation and stability through the shoulder girdle. This strength and stability enables the child to develop coordinated mobility throughout his body and to use his arms and hands for object exploration and manipulation. Stability in these areas, as well as in the head and neck, facilitates oral-motor, feeding, and expressive communication skills.

Areas of intervention could include the following:

- balance, equilibrium, and protective reactions
- vestibular functioning (i.e., the ability to orient yourself when you move your head or body; to maintain a stable position)
- muscle tone and strength
- joint and postural stability
- weight bearing, weight shifts, and trunk rotation
- sensory awareness and processing
- sensorimotor integration
- awareness of the body in space
- bilateral integration (being aware of and using both sides of the body in an integrated way)
- positioning and position transitions (e.g., from sit to stand)
- locomotion
- abdominal strength (These muscles are the central control area for postural stability, respiration, and breath support for speech.)

- respiration and breath control
- graded, controlled motor movement
- fine motor skills:
    feeding
    exploring the environment
    manipulation of objects and play
    self-help skills
    task performance and completion
    pre-academics (e.g., painting, cutting with scissors)
    academics (e.g., pencil grasp, copying)
- motor planning
- oral-motor skills
- perceptual motor skills

It's important to work closely with a pediatric physical therapist and/or occupational therapist on a team to facilitate normal skills, to improve the quality of these skills, and to decrease abnormal skills.

Chapter 6: Language Development

Language is the primary tool for learning about and acting on the world as well as for interacting with others. Comprehension and use of language requires the use of many skills, and there is an interrelationship among them. For example, the motor system is used for speech and language production as well as for moving through the environment and acting on it. Sensorimotor functioning and integration involve the ability to perceive information and then simultaneously process and organize from more than one sense. Language and cognitive functioning are so intertwined, that as increases are seen in one area, they are often mirrored in the other. All of these domains must develop appropriately and in coordination for the child to be able to interact, process, organize, clarify, recall, refine, and use information and language.

The individual with Down syndrome has difficulty with all aspects of communication, with some areas more impacted than others. Following are common questions and answers about language in Down syndrome. Intervention suggestions, including principles, strategies, and techniques, both general and those related to specific aspects of language development, are found in Chapter 7.

Do all individuals with Down syndrome achieve similar levels of language development?

There is great variance in overall communication skill development; however, there is greater potential for language learning and use than previously thought in the Down syndrome population. The overall level of language competence/achievement is dependent on:

- early and on-going appropriate stimulation and intervention
- the child's cognitive level
- motor skills
- motor-planning abilities
- sensorimotor skills
- the presence of sensory impairments
- health problems (e.g., heart defects, immunity problems, thyroid problems, seizures)

There is a range of language achievement in Down syndrome from those who are only able to express basic wants and needs to those who are able to comprehend and use fairly complex higher-level language. Those with more limited communication skills often benefit from a Total Communication approach using augmentative communication systems.

Many individuals with Down syndrome are capable of expanding their language skills well into their teens and early adulthood with continued therapy, education, and enrichment. To maximize a child's language ability, it is important to aggressively manage health issues (particularly hearing), begin intervention early, and continue at least through the teen years.

Do children with Down syndrome follow the same sequence of language development as their typically-developing peers?

There is some debate about this. One view is that Down syndrome language is not unique or deviant. These children acquire language skills later and at a slower rate, but go through the same developmental sequences as other children and follow the same rules that govern normal language development.

A second point of view holds that children with Down syndrome seem to have a unique pattern of development with greater difficulty mastering language in comparison to their other cognitive skills. There appear to be some specific difficulties that impede progress in learning language over and above the effects of a general cognitive delay. This view holds that children with Down syndrome do not merely have a slower version of normal language development, but actually have specific language learning deficits, particularly in the areas of vocabulary, morpho-syntax, language processing, and expressive language.

Overall, Down syndrome language learning appears to develop in a sequence similar to that of typically-developing children, but there are some significant differences including an unevenness in development with relative strengths and weaknesses. It appears to be appropriate to use a developmental progression for selecting targets for those with Down syndrome, but it's important to tailor language therapy to specific deficit areas for each child.

Which areas of communication development are relative strengths for the child with Down syndrome?

a. **Pre-language Skills**
   Many infants with Down syndrome demonstrate normal babbling, imitation, and vocalization behaviors. They are interested in early social games and spend about the same amount of time in this activity as other children.

b. **Play**
   The child with Down syndrome follows a similar sequence of development of play skills as her peers, with strengths in the social aspects of play. Symbolic play skills develop similarly to, although later than, other children. Those with higher cognitive skills tend to develop more mature and active play skills.

c. **Social Language**
   Pragmatics are a strength in comparison to other language skills. The social aspects of language need less intervention than other language skills. These children do well with most nonverbal social skills.

d. **Receptive Language**
   Language comprehension skills usually keep up with cognitive skills in the young child with Down syndrome. The child often has relative strengths in language comprehension, vocabulary comprehension, and grammar comprehension.

e. **Vocabulary**
   Semantics are a relative strength up to the age of 18 months with the ability to acquire words seemingly normal, though slow. Children with Down syndrome learn word meanings in the same way as their peers (e.g., using a fast-mapping system to acquire vocabulary).

f. **Expressive Language**
   There may not be a firm ceiling on expressive language development for the child with Down syndrome. Skills may increase with age with continued intervention and attention to health issues through early adulthood.

g. **Motor and Sensorimotor Skills**
   The child with Down syndrome has relative strengths in gestural communication, motor imitation, simple visual perception, and visual processing. Because of these strengths, the use of signing and written word appears to be particularly effective as learning strategies.

What differences are noted in the acquisition and use of language prerequisites in the young child with Down syndrome?

From an early age, there are noticeable differences in prelinguistic development in children with Down syndrome beyond those commonly associated with slow development. These differences are not solely related to cognitive deficits, but are also affected by brain differences, motor and sensorimotor difficulties, sensory impairments, low arousal, health problems, processing deficits, and poor muscle tone and strength including postural instability.

a. **Responsivity**

Infants with Down syndrome typically have a latency in response to others and the environment. They are slower to react/respond and are generally less aware, active, and reactive. This tendency to respond more slowly makes it difficult to develop early reciprocal nonverbal and communicative interactions and to learn from the environment. This impacts the child's learning throughout life.

b. **Visual Attention/Gaze**

Infants with Down syndrome demonstrate decreased visual awareness, visual attention, visual tracking, and eye contact. Gaze, an early form of communication and intent, is also difficult for these children. It develops more slowly and differs from other infants in flexibility and control. There is difficulty shifting attention between toys and people, and less sustained eye contact and referential eye contact (i.e., eye contact to the object or person that should be the subject of attention). They tend to spend much less time visually exploring their world and are more interested in and attentive to people rather than objects in their environment.

Infants with Down syndrome display difficulty with joint attention (i.e., the child and the adult attend to the same thing at the same time), an important contributor to cognitive and language development.

c. **Facial Expressions/Behavior**

Infants with Down syndrome are slow to develop a variety of facial expressions, have a reduced range of facial expressions, and demonstrate less intensity in their expressions and reactions. This makes it difficult for others to interpret the child's nonverbal communications. These infants also have difficulty reading the facial expressions of others which can lead to a breakdown in verbal and nonverbal exchanges.

d. **Vocalization**

In general, vocal development follows a similar, but delayed sequence to that of other children. The child with Down syndrome tends to vocalize less frequently, have a smaller sound inventory, takes longer to respond, and has difficulty with the turn-taking aspect of vocalizations. This causes her to be out of rhythm with her communicative partner. Frequently there is an imbalance of turns or one partner talks over the other.

e. **Babbling**

Although early babbling can be age-typical, reduplicated and variegated babbling are often delayed and less stable. The delayed development of competence with higher-level babbling skills can impact speech development by limiting practice with various sound combinations and sound sequences.

f. **Gestures**

Although it follows a similar sequence as that of other children, the development of gestures is delayed. Gesture can be a relative strength for children with Down syndrome in relation to other communication skills even though they often have difficulty coordinating gestures with eye gaze and/or vocalizations.

Signed communication becomes a strength for the child at the one- and two-word level, however many children with Down syndrome continue to use gestures to support communication rather than developing age-appropriate communication skills.

g. **Turn-taking**

Turn-taking forms the basis for all verbal and nonverbal communication exchanges and is critical for development of communication skills.

Children with Down syndrome are slow to develop turn-taking skills, although this improves with age. Their reciprocal interactions can be affected by:

- reduced alertness and attention
- a tendency to be less responsive and reactive
- poor initiation of turns
- difficulty with the timing and coordination of turn-taking
- a delay in response time
- responses which are more difficult to read
- difficulty developing and using a reliable signaling system
- an imbalance in turn-taking with the child responding in an inconsistent manner
- others not giving the child time to respond and take her turn in the exchange

What is the basis for communication deficits in Down syndrome?

a. Brain Differences
The brain in children with Down syndrome tends to be smaller in size and weight than that of similar-aged peers. There are also differences in brain growth and development, myelinization of the central nervous system, communication between the hemispheres/lobes of the brain, the neurotransmitter system, the number of neurons and synaptic connections, cerebral specialization, and cellular development.

b. Cognitive Deficits
Because of mental retardation along with significant differences in neurological development, children with Down syndrome have more difficulty with language than others with similar cognitive abilities. All areas of communication are impacted.

c. Sensory Impairments
Many children with Down syndrome have recurring otitis media, hearing loss, and problems with wax impaction. Middle ear problems tend to be bilateral and chronic. Most individuals with Down syndrome demonstrate conductive and/or sensorineural hearing deficits over time.

Many children with Down syndrome also have visual impairments, difficulty with tactile and proprioceptive awareness and sensitivity, deficits in sensory regulation and integration, and difficulty with sensorimotor skills.

d. Processing Deficits
These children have difficulty receiving and processing sensory information from individual modalities as well as difficulty integrating sensory information from more than one sense at a time. Visual processing skills are much stronger than auditory processing abilities, which are often significantly impaired.

Auditory processing problems affect the whole communication profile of individuals with Down syndrome. They have difficulty with attention and vigilance, need more time to process information, and are slower to respond. They have difficulty with auditory reception, long- and short-term memory, selective attention, sequential information, word retrieval, and analysis and synthesis. There is also decreased processing of proprioceptive and tactile input.

A key contributor to language deficits in the Down syndrome population appears to be a limited auditory short-term memory. This especially impedes expressive language and morpho-syntax skill development.

e. Motor Delays
Delays in motor skill development can affect the child's perception and knowledge of the world and her ability to explore and interact with the environment and others. This in turn affects language development, particularly early vocabulary and concept development. Delays in motor skills, low tone, and postural instability also affect the child's ability to use expressive language, whether spoken or signed.

Low tone, muscle weakness, instability of the trunk and shoulder girdle, inadequate motor organization, motor planning difficulties, and poor oral-motor skills all contribute to difficulty with communication skills, particularly with expressive language and speech.

What patterns are present in play development in the child with Down syndrome?

Play is how children learn about their world. Play is important for developing engagement, attention, and reciprocation; and provides an environment for learning cognitive and language skills. Piaget saw play as closely associated with the growth of intelligence. It allows children to acquire and practice new skills and to consolidate learning.

A child's level of play and the quality of her play generally reflect developmental and language levels. Children who demonstrate pre-linguistic behaviors also demonstrate pre-symbolic play behaviors. Children who are at a one-word utterance stage of development use single schemes in their play. When children are able to combine words in their utterances, they generally are able to combine play schemes.

Children with Down syndrome have delays in the acquisition of various play skills, although the social aspects of play typically are strengths for them. They tend to follow the same developmental sequences as their peers, but at a slower rate with a wider range of abilities. They tend to experience a diminished range and variety of interactional play. A major goal for children with Down syndrome is to help them develop independent and interactive play.

There are some distinctive characteristics found in the play of children with Down syndrome. A major characteristic during play (and learning) is a tendency toward passivity and a lack of responsiveness. These children tend to be "watchers" rather than "doers" during play, spending longer periods of passive watching than their peers. They make fewer requests, explore their environment and toys less, and are slower to interact with objects, people, and the environment. Because they are slower in their processing and responses, the movement in the play may pass too quickly for them to actively participate. The child with Down syndrome may not take a turn so there is an imbalance in turns with the play partner, or the partner may do the child's part as well as her own. The child may need a verbal or physical prompt to get started and to continue interactive play and may need modeling of new ways to play.

Another characteristic is a lack of change and creativity in play with a tendency toward repetitive play. The child may have difficulty attending to toys and her attention may be easily diverted during play. She may demonstrate a limited number of schemes for acting on objects so that she often plays with the same objects in the same way rather than expanding her play schemes or using novel ones. She may reject new schemes by refusing them or losing interest. There is a tendency to stay with familiar toys and to reject mastery-type toys (e.g., puzzles, shape ball), even those the child could be successful with. The child with Down syndrome also demonstrates a delay in using two objects together in play. This limits the child's development of new schemes and learning about the world around her. These tendencies can be related to motor-planning difficulties as well as to cognitive deficits.

Even though social aspects of play are relative strengths, many with Down syndrome tend not to engage others in play, even at early stages using showing, giving, and turn-taking behaviors. This limits their play opportunities. They may become isolated because of their limited ability to use language during play to interact, to direct, and to expand play schemes and scenarios.

What other difficulties in communication are noted in Down syndrome?

Individuals with Down syndrome have impairments at all levels of communication. Pueschel (1992) states that they often have greater difficulty with language than other mentally handicapped individuals with similar cognitive abilities.

a. **Asynchrony of Development**
   Asynchrony of language skill development is a major characteristic seen in Down syndrome. Some language skills are more delayed than others.

   • Comprehension is often commensurate with mental ability in young children while spoken vocabulary and syntax lag behind.

- Overall communication skills are greater than verbal skills due to higher personal and social skills than cognitive and expressive language skills.

- Expressive skills are quite delayed in relation to receptive skills, particularly morpho-syntactic skills. Comprehension is more advanced than production skills.

- Gestural communication is a relative strength in comparison to speech and expressive language skills, especially during the preschool years.

- Visual skills are stronger than auditory skills with a faster reaction time to visual signals. Visual processing skills are much higher than auditory.

- Concrete language skills are stronger than abstract language and thinking skills.

- Expressive language skills become relatively weaker over time, and as the child's mental age increases, her expressive skills often don't keep up.

b. **Instability of Language Learning**

An instability in language learning and skill acquisition is typical in the Down syndrome population. It can be due to incomplete reception and processing of information; partial learning; a lack of practice of skills; a lack of integration of new information and skills; loss of old skills; and difficulty with organization, memory, awareness, retrieval, processing, generalization and consolidation of learned information.

c. **Reduced Motivation to Communicate**

It's often difficult to determine the child's true communication abilities because of a reduced motivation to communicate and perform. This may arise from the child's difficulty in keeping up with the conversation due to language deficits or her experience with communicative failure which leads her to believe that her communications will be misunderstood. Her poor timing and difficulty with reciprocity in communicating may also lead to repeated communication failures. This is complicated by a tendency to miss conversational cues due to reduced eye contact and attention to the partner's message. The child may be more motivated to communicate in social settings or during social routines.

The child's reduced motivation to communicate may be manifested in the following ways:

- a pattern of watching rather than doing; a tendency to be a passive participant and learner
- inattentiveness to verbal tasks and exchanges
- low task vigilance and persistence
- refusal or avoidance
- use of manipulative behaviors

d. **Vocabulary Development**

Children with Down syndrome learn word meanings in the same way as other children, but they learn new words and expand their total vocabulary at a slower rate. Their relative skill with vocabulary tends to decline with age and by 18 months they have a smaller overall vocabulary than other children. Their vocabulary ends up being smaller than would be expected in relation to cognitive development. Vocabulary does not increase as fast as it should in relation to the child's mental age.

The age of rapid acceleration of vocabulary also differs in the Down syndrome and typical populations. Children with Down syndrome often don't go through a vocabulary spurt at 18 months, or when they have 20–50 words, as do other children. Instead, they begin this rapid vocabulary growth at a much later age when they have approximately twice the number of words as other children.

Expressively, the child with Down syndrome uses significantly fewer spoken words than typically-developing children of the same mental age. When both spoken and signed words are counted, however, the child with Down syndrome often uses the same number of lexicon items as her peers, although the signed and spoken vocabulary are often made up of different words.

e. **Expressive Language**

Developmental Milestones for Expressive Language in Children with Down Syndrome Compared to Their Typically-Developing Peers		
	Down Syndrome	Typically Developing
first words	2-5 years	12 months
first 10 words	27 months	15 months
use of 18 words	3 years	18 months
vocabulary spurt	30 months	18 months
two-word phrases	36-48 months	19-22 months
4 years	1.5 MLU	4.5 MLU
6 years	3.5 MLU	5+ MLU
15 years	5+ MLU	

f. **MLU from Two-Word to Multi-Word Utterances**
Children with Down syndrome tend to use the same range of two-word constructions as typically-developing children, but have a larger single word vocabulary when they begin to put two words together (about 100 words rather than 50 as for other children). In other words, they have more words before they start to combine them than other children.

Children with Down syndrome have a shorter mean length of utterance (MLU) than same-aged peers. Many reach the two-word utterance stage between the ages of 3 and 4, although some are later. MLU tends to increase with age until early adolescence. Some young adults continue to expand their length of utterance.

The slowness and limitation in MLU development in children with Down syndrome is directly related to difficulties with morpho-syntax and memory skills. They have increasing difficulty as they reach the 2 ½ to 3 ½ word utterance level (Brown's Stage III).

At Stage III, children begin to use grammatical structures. Earlier stages were characterized by basic word order and semantic relations. At Stage III, grammar becomes increasingly challenging for the child with Down syndrome and there is significant difficulty from the three-word utterance level on. They have difficulty in the ability to organize the sequence of words and to combine words syntactically to make longer sentences. For the children with Down syndrome who progress beyond Stage III, there can be a dramatic increase in MLU and grammatical complexity.

g. **Morpho-Syntax**
Individuals with Down syndrome have greater difficulty with morphology and syntax than other aspects of language, probably because it is more abstract, complex, and involves longer utterances. Poor short-term memory, difficulty with speech intelligibility, auditory processing deficits, motor-planning deficits, and difficulty with breath control for speech may contribute to this difficulty.

Difficulty with speech intelligibility appears to affect sentence production even in early childhood. The child may learn to use shorter, less grammatically complex utterances in order to be understood. This often becomes a life-long pattern of sacrificing syntax for intelligibility.

Children with Down syndrome appear to have more difficulty with both receptive and expressive syntax than others with the same mental age. They follow the same pattern of development as other children but progress much slower and reach lower levels. They tend to produce as many utterances as other children but their language has fewer of Brown's Stage III and IV structures. They show increasing difficulty with morpho-syntactic development beyond the ages of 3-4 as their skills don't keep pace with their cognitive development and are less complex for their developmental level.

Their growth in syntax may occur in spurts with long plateaus over childhood and adolescence until they reach an average length of utterance of four words. Some develop more complex syntactic structures and the use of lengthy utterances. They tend to use vocabulary strategies such as key words to convey meaning rather than using morphological and syntactical structures (e.g., they use the terms "yesterday/today/tomorrow" to denote verb tense, but do not actually use the verb tenses: "I go to the store yesterday.").

How adults communicate with the child could contribute to her difficulty in learning morphology and syntax. There is a tendency for adults to ask closed questions, to prompt and fill in for the child, to answer for the child, to interpret the child's utterances to others, and to not give the child enough time to formulate a response. This tendency may affect the child's ability to learn and generate longer and more complex utterances.

h. **Pragmatics**
This is an area of relative strength, particularly for the younger child. A deceleration is often seen with age because later social skills are dependent on language. Increasing pragmatic deficits may be manifested as difficulty with:

- attending skills and eye contact
- initiating interaction
- verbal and nonverbal requesting behavior
- topic selection and maintenance
- turn-taking
- a latency in response time
- asking and responding to questions
- asking appropriate questions and making appropriate statements
- asking for and making clarifications and repairs
- interpreting social cues and reading facial expressions
- using polite conversation forms for softening requests and statements
- proxemics (i.e., how close to stand to another person, when to make physical contacts such as hugging)
- taking the listener's knowledge and perspective into account

i. **Conversational Pragmatics**
The communications of those with Down syndrome can cover a wide range of topics, but conversations typically are short because they may not take turns

and they may lack relevant knowledge to keep the conversation going. They may respond to questions but not ask them to keep the conversation going. They respond less contingently and have a timing problem when interacting (e.g., slow processing, reacting, and responding). There is a tendency to use concrete vocabulary and to talk about the here-and-now rather than about remote events.

Adolescents and adults often have difficulty being understood by their conversational partners due to poor intelligibility and a lack of repair strategies. In addition, they tend to have difficulty reading the facial expressions of others, a deficit compounded by poor eye contact. They may experience social isolation partly as a result of a lack of adequate language and conversational skills.

j. **Processing**
Individuals with Down syndrome often have significant difficulty with processing skills, particularly auditory processing. They also have difficulty processing and integrating information from more than one sense at a time. Poor processing affects language comprehension and production. Specific processing deficits may include:

- decreased attention span and low reactivity
- slow orienting to auditory information
- the need for more time to process information and respond
- difficulty with all aspects of auditory processing, particularly sequential and short-term memory
- frequent need for repetition of instruction, questions, etc.
- difficulty with visual sequential memory
- decreased processing of proprioceptive and tactile input
- difficulty organizing and retrieving information
- difficulty processing speech—poor reception and discrimination of speech (i.e., hearing the differences in words)
- difficulty dealing with complex or multiple sensory stimuli

What communication characteristics are seen in the older Down syndrome population?

As they get older, there appear to be increasing deficits in language and communication skills relative to other abilities. Teens and adults show language levels lower than would be expected in comparison to their cognitive development. However, they often can show gains with continued intervention through early adulthood. Their communications may be characterized by:

- immature grammar skills
- frequent use of social conversational routines or stereotypical expressions in their speech
- a tendency to use short telegraphic utterances which may contain only the key words
- continued difficulty with processing information
- continued difficulty with speech intelligibility (i.e., immature phonological and articulatory patterns)
- decreased intelligibility with the use of longer and more complex utterances
- social, community, and work success impeded by communication deficits
- inconsistency in communication performance
- dementia, associated with Alzheimer's, in a portion of the population as they age (There seems to be a lengthy period between the onset of Alzheimer's and the onset of dementia.)

What behaviors may be noted secondary to communication difficulty in Down syndrome?

Individuals with Down syndrome often experience communication failure resulting in communication avoidance. This may be manifested by:

- reduced attending, eye contact, and joint attention
- reduced interest/motivation
- reluctance to use communication to meet their needs
- attempts to conform behaviorally without fully processing or using active communication
- reluctance to request information
- failure by default (i.e., a tendency to give up rather than attempting conversation or conversational repairs)
- reluctance to attempt or to repeat attempts
- verbal or task avoidance
- manipulative behaviors
- passivity (i.e., looking rather than doing or communicating)
- acting out, refusal, or reduced cooperation

Chapter 7: Language Intervention

The more that is done to overcome language delay and speech difficulty, the better equipped the individual with Down syndrome will be to function independently. This chapter addresses language intervention principles and specific strategies for those principles. Because of the interrelation between language and cognition, it is important to read Chapter 3 in conjunction with this one. Specific information about speech development and use is found in Chapter 8.

It is critical that intervention begins early, and that speech-language therapy continues at least through the teen years. In later adulthood, a portion of those with Down syndrome develop Alzheimer's-type dementia and may benefit from therapy to enhance and augment memory skills.

General Principles of Intervention

1. Begin by assessing capabilities as well as weaknesses, using formal and informal measures as well as observations and interviews of family members and teachers. Then manipulate the environment to support the child's strengths and to work around his weaknesses.

2. Select goals and objectives based on identification of functional skills and assessment findings. Arrange them in an intervention hierarchy. Although children with Down syndrome have general characteristics in common, therapy should be planned to meet the needs of the individual child. No one plan, or cookbook approach, is going to meet the needs of all children. Each child needs to move at his own pace toward goals that are appropriate for his unique combination of abilities and differences. Select goals that:

   • are developmentally appropriate
   • are functional
   • are sequential (i.e., steps to master a task)
   • develop prerequisite skills
   • increase communication skills

3. Use teaching strategies such as the following that lead to success.

   • Increase auditory and visual attention.
   • Use the visual channel as much as possible to augment and help overcome auditory processing deficits. Visual stimuli can be used to increase comprehension as well as for cueing new expressive language structures. Visual input may include pictures, photos, written word, visual symbols, gestures, and/or sign.
   • Build on what the child can do. Gradually increase the complexity of the tasks.
   • Incorporate the child's areas of interest.
   • Progress from skills within the child's repertoire to novel ones; progress from immediate to delayed imitation.

- Use error-free learning initially to teach new skills (i.e., give the child maximum cues so he cannot make a mistake, like limiting the number of choices available or physically guiding the child using hand-over-hand).
- Choose behaviors easy for the child to perform.

4. Use movement and positioning to help facilitate muscle tone and respiration/phonation, to regulate alertness, and to facilitate language learning and use.

5. Begin intervention early to help the child develop prerequisite skills for learning and using language.

6. Interact with and talk to individuals with Down syndrome in effective ways.

   - Be alert to the child's means of engaging others (e.g., fleeting eye contact, a vocalization, a gesture).
   - Be responsive and treat the child as an active learning partner, but don't be too quick to respond or the child won't have a reason to communicate.
   - Give the child time to initiate as well as to respond.
   - Monitor the number of directives and questions used. Too frequent use can adversely affect the child's spontaneous verbal output.
   - Use functional tasks, daily activities, routines, and play to build in practice and carryover of new skills.
   - Slow the rate of presentation to the child and reduce distractors.
   - Use paralinguistic cues such as varying the rhythm, stress, inflection, pitch, and loudness to help gain and maintain the child's attention.
   - Give specific feedback and reinforcement to the child.

7. Teach parents and others in the child's environment how to facilitate communication skills. Be supportive of the parents and others in their efforts.

   - Give information about general development, health issues, and development of communication skills in children with Down syndrome.
   - Give strategies for helping the child develop language as well as the prerequisite skills needed for language.
   - Explain the developmental sequence of communication skills in the typical and Down syndrome populations.
   - Demonstrate teaching techniques as well as cueing techniques.
   - Teach to be aware of and to respond to all types of communications.
   - Teach not to overwhelm the child with too much physical or verbal stimulation, and to give the child time to initiate and respond.
   - Involve the whole family, including siblings, grandparents, aunts and uncles, etc.

8. Engage the child to foster learning and interaction (e.g., get the child's interest; have fun with him).

   - Use child-centered therapy (for young children, it's play-based).
   - Get down to the child's level (e.g., floor play, on lap, face-to-face).
   - Let the child initiate an activity or topic, then follow the child's lead.
   - Imitate the child's behavior or verbalization.
   - Match the child's developmental level.
   - Use the child's emotions as the starting point for every interaction.
   - Use objects/events the child is interested in. Use novel objects, movement, and change to entice the child into engagement.
   - Include play activities that parallel home routines.

9. Use play to encourage exploration and to facilitate language learning and use. When the child is focused on toys and action, verbalizations often occur spontaneously.

10. Expect the child to communicate.

    - Encourage more opportunities for the child to initiate communication so he becomes a more active and less reactive communicator.
    - Use interrupted chains in routine activities to encourage initiation (e.g., when preparing the bath, "forget" part of the sequence as the child watches or helps [put in the bath toys, but forget

the water]; tell the child his bath is ready; look expectantly at him or cue him that you are waiting for him to say something).
- Encourage a response by letting the child know you expect one.
- Interrupt behavior chains and require a response.
- Prompt, pause, and look expectantly.
- Give verbal prompts.

11. Arrange the environment to facilitate turn-taking, to keep the interchange going, or to facilitate a response. Be sure to respond to the child's looking, reaching, pointing, verbalizing, gesturing, and signing. Use balanced turns with neither partner dominating. Match actions and communications to the child's level, then expand them.

    Set up communication-demand situations. Sabotage the environment by:

    - delaying responding to a request; misunderstanding the communication, request, or question; giving the wrong item; acting confused
    - presenting favorite objects just out of the child's reach
    - structuring situations where the child needs adult assistance to obtain a desired object, or having necessary parts or objects missing
    - interrupting at critical moments during routines or activities, waiting, and looking expectantly for the child to communicate
    - stopping an activity the child wants to continue and delaying continuation until he communicates
    - playing obstructively by getting in the child's way to create an interaction

12. Keep the interactions going. Let the child know he is expected to participate in the conversation. Establish a reciprocal, rather than a dead-end, contact by:

    - responding to the message
    - cueing the child to respond
    - avoiding close-ended questions and comments
    - not dominating the interaction
    - holding out for a better turn (i.e., don't give what he wants too quickly)

13. Assign communicative meaning. Act as if the child communicated so you can shape responses into language. Pair his current vocalizations and verbalizations with actions, objects, people, and routines, making them meaningful communications (e.g., the child produces a sequence of syllables [babbling] while looking at a ball. The adult provides words and meaning, "Ball. That's a ball. Do you want the ball?" and gives the ball to the child).

14. Establish social and joint action routines (i.e., sequences of actions to make up a routine such as the steps used during dressing) to teach language through social experiences. Children with Down syndrome may be more motivated to learn communication in social settings or during social routines. Routines allow the child to anticipate what will happen next and to increase opportunities for practice and use of language in natural settings. To establish routines:

    - use highly motivating experiences
    - make learning into games and positive social interactions
    - organize daily activities into regular, sequential experiences/formats to help the child learn and anticipate sequences of behavior
    - embed language targets into familiar scripts and routines
    - begin with existing routines to provide consistency and predictability
    - interrupt routine sequences to create a reason to communicate and to prompt the use of spontaneous language
    - teach and practice new routines
    - use different types of routines and joint action routines such as social games, songs, fingerplays, social amenities, and daily caregiving activities (e.g., toileting, dressing, bathing)

15. Use augmentative communication for receptive and expressive learning and use. The child can use it to supplement spoken language as needed to help others understand him.

    - Total Communication can help the child transition to speech while providing a system for him to express new skills, wants, and needs. It also is useful as a strategy for teaching language.

- Photo and picture albums or books with vocabulary Items or syntax structures are useful augmentative tools to help the child practice language targets or to help him convey or clarify his messages.

- Computers are useful because they are visual, and their speed, content, level of input, and task difficulty can all be controlled. They allow for repeated practice in a predictable way.

16. Use peer interaction where other children serve as models and conversational partners.

17. Use direct teaching for language skills not in the child's repertoire. Children with Down syndrome need direct instruction to build language skills because they don't learn as readily from incidental teaching as others. They need controlled, structured, and multiple exposure to language targets. Naturalistic teaching doesn't provide as many of these structured exposures.

    - Use direct teaching for all areas of communication including vocabulary, pragmatic, processing, and morphosyntactic skills.
    - Emphasize attention, listening, and processing.
    - Model many examples of the target; repetition is important.
    - Reduce distracters and control variables; gradually add new elements.
    - Provide repeated practice and drill. Children with Down syndrome need repetitive practice in order to move to a more automatic level of learning and production.
    - Teach at or slightly above the child's level.
    - Use teaching strategies that provide learning experiences rather than asking questions to determine the child's knowledge (i.e., teaching, not testing).

18. Use reinforcement to encourage learning.

19. Use a variety of therapy strategies and techniques to teach language such as:

- chaining (a type of shaping)
    - forward – teach the first unit in a sequence first
    - backward – teach the last unit in a sequence first
    - interrupted chains
- clarifying words, statements, requests, and questions that the child doesn't seem to understand
- using cues and prompts
- establish a cueing hierarchy – most to least assistance
    - physical prompt (e.g., partial physical guidance; full physical guidance)
    - model
    - verbal cue
- providing drill and repetitive practice
- eliciting receptive and expressive responses with the same task (e.g., saying "Show me" followed by "What did you get?"). This facilitates focused attention and active learning.
- embedding language into social routines/scripts
- expanding the child's utterances
- extending by responding to the child's utterance with a related one
- fading (i.e., gradually reducing the level of cueing or prompting)
- giving input to the child's sensory, cognitive, and motor systems to facilitate alertness, responsivity, cooperation, and performance
- having the child imitate the adult's model or having the adult imitate the child and then encouraging the child to imitate back
- using incomplete sentences to elicit new vocabulary and increase spontaneous language
- making a selection when given a choice of items, activities, etc.
- matching the child's level of performance or providing activities that are slightly above his level
- modeling language targets
- providing multisensory cueing
- pausing (i.e., waiting; looking expectantly for a turn or a response)
- using prosody variations (e.g., loudness, pitch, intonational contours) to stress and call the child's attention to target language elements
- questioning with modeled answers

- recasting for communication repairs (i.e., saying something a different way to make the meaning clearer)
- rephrasing/restating directions, questions, or the child's utterance
- using scripts and carrier phrases
- having the child finish sentences (e.g., "The dog is _____.")
- shaping (i.e., breaking a task into small sequential steps, each of which is a closer approximation to the target behavior)

20. Facilitate generalization of language skills. Once the child demonstrates the target language skill in structured settings, use incidental teaching to help the child generalize.

   - Teach language in the context of meaningful use and in meaningful activities.
   - Teach multiple examples.
   - Teach the skill in its natural setting.
   - Use a variety of objects/activities in teaching.
   - Teach the skill in different settings.
   - Use different people in teaching.
   - Give lots of opportunities for language practice.
   - Reward the use of language.
   - Create opportunities for language by giving the child a need to communicate.

21. Work on speech and language skills at the same time. When working on a word production, also use it for different functions such as to request or comment.

22. Teach some carrier phrases and automatic speech so children with limited verbal skills have an immediate way to communicate and interact. Target frequently occurring words and phrases in the child's environment to facilitate conversation initiation.

Early Communication Strategies

Facilitate development of early cognitive skills, prerequisite skills, and early language skills to enhance the child's general readiness for communication and learning. These include:

Awareness of Sound and Sound Localization

Stimulate awareness and localization of sound by:

- calling the child's attention to sounds that occur in familiar routines (e.g., doorbell ringing, phone ringing)
- pairing a specific event or activity with a sound (e.g., running bath water and getting in the tub)
- pairing the sound with a visual model (e.g., having the child look at a rattle as you shake it)
- calling to the child or calling the child's name
- using toys that make sounds
- having people and/or toys in different places around the room make noises
- showing the child two objects, using one to make a sound, and prompting the child to look toward it or select it

Visual Attention

This includes gaze/reciprocal gaze, diverted gaze (e.g., looking at or toward a named object or person), and visual tracking. To facilitate:

- use toys or objects with interesting actions (e.g., wind-up toys, toys that light up or make noise)
- use a flashlight or interesting toy near the adult's face to gain the child's attention
- use balloons and bubbles
- use pull-toys and move them slowly across the child's line of vision
- use a verbal or physical prompt such as "Look here," or "Look at the _____"

Object Permanence

Object permanence is the knowledge that an object exists, even when it is out of sight. This is related to word knowledge and use. To facilitate:

- put an object in front of the child and partially cover it while he's watching
- put an object in front of the child and cover it completely while he's watching; then prompt him to find the object
- hide an object under one of two covers and prompt the child to find it

- drop a toy or a piece of food and have the child look for it
- play "Peek-a-boo"

Means to an End, Cause and Effect, and Causality

These involve the ability to solve problems mentally and to understand that one's behavior can affect and be affected by others. To facilitate:

- use daily activities such as turning on the water faucet, pushing a doorbell, or using a switch to turn the lights on
- use cause-and-effect toys such as a busy box, push 'n go toys, or a wind-up music box
- use toys that require an adult's help to activate
- use toys with on-off switches
- use cause-and-effect software on the computer (e.g., when the child pushes a key on the keyboard or touches the computer screen, a character moves on the screen)

Tool Use

Stimulate the early use of tools by:

- helping the child pull a string to bring a toy closer to him
- placing a toy on the child's blanket and helping him pull it toward himself
- using eating utensils to pick up food or to get food out of a jar
- using markers and crayons
- using toys that involve early "tools" such as a hammer and pegs, tongs to pick up cotton balls, or a xylophone and stick

Joint Attention and Interaction

In order to develop language, a child must develop joint attention (i.e., both the child and the adult are paying attention to the same thing) and interaction. Once these are established, begin working on turn-taking skills since the development of all of these skills overlap. To facilitate:

- give the child time to orient and process

- position the child so he has maximum ability to focus on the object, person, or activity
- remove distractions from the environment and use a limited number of toys to keep the child focused
- follow the child's lead; begin by attending to what the child attends to
- imitate what the child is doing
- gradually enter the child's play until both you and the child are playing jointly with the same toys
- use interesting or novel objects that will capture the child's attention such as ones that are moveable, have multiple parts, or have interesting actions or features
- give or offer the child a toy
- play social games (e.g., "Peek-a-boo") and use fingerplays
- use verbal or physical prompts to get the child to look at or toward a person or object. Let the child know what you want him to attend to.
- stop interfering behaviors (e.g., self-stimulation, perseverative behaviors)
- reward the child for paying attention using natural rewards (i.e., If he looks at a toy, he gets the toy.)

Turn-taking

Turn-taking is an early pragmatic skill on which all communication is based. Children typically develop turn-taking first with actions, then with vocalizations and verbalizations. Once turn-taking has been established, begin working on direct imitation. The development of turn-taking and imitation skills is very interrelated. The following strategies will help facilitate turn-taking and imitation skills.

Establish turn-taking with actions.
- Begin by imitating the child's actions (i.e., the first turn is the adult's response to the child's actions). After the child performs an action on a toy or object, take it, and repeat the action. Return the toy to the child, look expectantly, and wait for him to take a turn.
- Prompt the child to take a turn as needed.
- Match actions to the child's actions and take balanced turns.
- Use interesting, developmentally-appropriate toys and actions.
- Choose actions that are easy for the child to perform.

- Demonstrate an activity and give the child the toy or object to take a turn.
- Request a turn, take the turn, give the object back to the child, and prompt him to take a turn by saying, "Your turn."
- Start with give-and-take or exchange toys such as push 'n go vehicles (i.e., toys that you push down on the top and then let go so they automatically move forward).
- Use put-in/take-out (e.g., blocks/basket), put-on/take-off (e.g., stacking rings), throw/catch (e.g., balls), and push/pull activities (e.g., push 'n go vehicles, busy boxes).

Follow the same sequence for establishing turn-taking with vocalizations and verbalizations.
- Imitate the child's vocalizations, look expectantly, wait for his turn, give verbal prompts to take a turn.
- Use environmental sounds while playing (e.g., car sounds), waiting for a response, or requesting a response.
- When the child makes sounds, make a sound in response. (It does not have to be the same sound; this is turn-taking, not imitation.)

Keep the interchange going.
- Keep the turns short and simple and similar to the child's.
- Gradually increase the number of turns taken.
- Match the child's level.
- Pause to give the child time to respond and look expectantly.
- If waiting doesn't work, prompt or signal the child to take a turn.
- Be responsive to the child. Don't rush him, but wait, pause, and look for continued action or communication that can be shaped into a turn.

Expand or model better turns.
- Imitate and expand the child's turn by adding one small step at a time.
- Change one element of the child's turn. (e.g., The child is dropping blocks on the floor. On your turn, drop a block in a container. If the child pats a car, you push it.)

Establish routines within daily activities so the child can predict and know how and when to react.

Imitation

Begin with immediate, then delayed or deferred imitation; first with actions, then vocalizations and verbalizations.

(See turn-taking strategies on pages 62-63 in addition to the strategies below.)

- Give the child time to process the action or verbal model and then imitate it; frequently there is a latency in response time.

- Facilitate imitation of gestures and actions.
  - ▸ Initially, imitate the child's action and see if he'll imitate in return. Use physical or verbal prompts.
  - ▸ Encourage the child to imitate simple actions and gestures (e.g., "So Big," "Pat-a-Cake," pushing a toy car).
  - ▸ Wait, pause, look expectantly, cue, and prompt the child to respond.
  - ▸ When the child imitates simple familiar actions freely, make a small change and encourage him to imitate.
  - ▸ If the child doesn't imitate, repeat the behavior and verbal cue, then physically prompt the child. Give verbal reinforcement.
  - ▸ Introduce a novel action and encourage the child to imitate.
  - ▸ Chain imitation turns together, then expand the child's repertoire by making a change.
  - ▸ Introduce simple fingerplays.

- Facilitate imitation of vocalizations (e.g., cooing, "raspberries") and verbalizations (e.g., actual speech sounds).
  - ▸ Follow the same sequence as used for actions.
  - ▸ Introduce different sounds such as sound effects, animal sounds, environmental sounds, non-speech sounds, and speech sounds for imitation.
  - ▸ Combine motor movements and sounds (e.g., make a sound as you jump) as movement can stimulate sound production.
  - ▸ Introduce a sound associated with an action during play (e.g., "boom" as you knock down blocks) and cue the child to imitate.

▸ Introduce a sound associated with an object or picture (e.g., "ba" for "bottle," "ma" for "Mama").

▸ When the child begins imitating, interrupt play and ask for an imitation to continue the activity or to get more of a desired object.

▸ Have the child imitate isolated vowels and consonants, and then use them in real situations (e.g., "mmmm" for something good to eat).

• Make imitation activities or games part of the daily routine.

Early Nonverbal Communication

Nonverbal communication includes any early vocal, nonverbal, or gestural pragmatic signal. This may include pointing, reaching, tugging or pulling at an adult; directed eye movements toward a desired object; turn-taking; vocalizing; patting; waving; or shaking the head for a *yes-no* response. Intervention strategies include the following:

1. Shape any looking, vocalizing, movement, or gesture into a signal by assigning meaning to it.

2. Establish a relationship between the signal (the child's nonverbal communication) and your response (e.g., the child puts his arms up and you pick him up).

3. Respond equally to gestures and vocalizations.

4. Arrange the environment so the child has to use a variety of nonverbal communications to get what he wants.

5. Start with simple gestures that can have communication meaning (e.g., reaching toward a desired object).

6. Encourage a variety of pragmatic functions and intentions:

   • giving (i.e., using toys and objects that encourage give-and-take exchanges like a ball for throw and catch, push 'n go vehicles, or toys that need an adult to activate)

   • commenting/showing/pointing (e.g., put interesting toys/objects in a bag or box for the child to take out, prompting him to show them). Do actions that encourage a response such as dropping something on the floor, turning the lights off, or wearing a funny hat or a clown nose.

   • requesting (i.e., engineer the environment so the child has to signal for an object or action; or for more of the action or object)

   • protesting/rejecting (i.e., give a choice between two objects, with one the child obviously won't want. Give him the least desirable object and wait for a response; prompt as needed.)

   • greeting (e.g., "Hi," "Bye," "Thank you," and "Please.") Model the greeting and pair with a gesture or sign. Give social rewards for a response.

   • making choices

     ▸ use desirable or favorite activities and objects

     ▸ limit the choices

     ▸ use choices that are visible

     ▸ accept any mode of making a choice such as a gaze, touch, point, reach, gesture, vocalization

     ▸ act as if the child had made a choice (i.e., If the child looks at an object, give it along with verbal praise for making a choice)

     ▸ reward immediately with the activity or object

7. Use peer modeling.

8. Expand to new objects, activities, people, settings, photos, pictures with written word, and signs. Incorporate them into daily routines and social activities.

Play Skill Strategies

Facilitate play skills in the child with Down syndrome. Play typically develops in the following sequence:

1. The child acts on single objects, one scheme per object, then on a variety of schemes with that object. (Early schemes may include shake, bang, grasp-and-release, and put-in/take-out behaviors.)

2. The child performs a variety of schemes for acting on various objects (e.g., uses a spoon to bang or to offer a bite to Mom; uses a cup in the bathtub to fill, pour, and drink from).

3. The child plays with single objects in a functional way, then combinations of objects (e.g., expands from rocking a baby doll to using a blanket with the doll to put it to bed).

4. The child imitates daily activities, building to increasingly complex play schemes incorporating more objects.

5. The child uses representational play (e.g., lines up blocks on the floor to make a road or train track).

6. The child uses creative play (e.g., recreates familiar themes like pretending to be a doctor).

7. The child uses imaginative play (e.g., creates new scenarios).

8. The child plays games with rules.

To facilitate play skills:

- have developmentally-appropriate toys available and make the interactions fun and interactive
- use toys the child has an interest in
- reduce distracters and start with a limited number of toys and choices
- use turn-taking toys to facilitate interactions; prompt the child to take his turn
- use toys that can be used in different ways or have multiples uses
- facilitate joint attention; joint focus on play objects and activities
- match and balance play so that the adult is not directing or dominating
- use physical prompts as needed to get the child started, to get him to take his turn, and to show him new ways to play
- move at the child's pace; allow him to have a range of experiences
- start with one toy and model a scheme for acting on it (e.g., Give the object to the child and prompt him to use it. You can also follow his lead, and imitate his schemes for acting on the object.)

- introduce new toys or objects and model a single scheme for each
- introduce new schemes for acting on a familiar toy (e.g., use a doll to hug, kiss, rock, put in bed, or wash). Keep these simple, introducing one or two schemes at a time. Gradually expand until the child can do multiple actions with a toy.
- begin to combine objects in play, starting with two and gradually expanding to more
- play with toys that reflect real-life activities; use realistic props in play
- teach the child to play in different ways with different objects
- set up play scenarios in routines (e.g., putting a doll to bed) and practice them
- add new actions and props as the routines become more familiar
- use techniques such as:
  modeling, prompting, and cueing
  imitating and turn-taking
  shaping behaviors
  chaining and interrupted chains
  using social routines and scripts
- expand scenarios to introduce higher levels of play such as creative play
- introduce games with simple rules

Receptive Language Strategies

Generally, children with Down syndrome will learn receptive language skills in the same sequence as other children, but they will achieve these skills at a lower level and at later ages. They need more practice and direct teaching to learn language and it often takes them longer to consolidate and integrate new information and skills.

These children need multiple experiences and many repetitions of target language structures in order to learn them, although if the child is bombarded with too much stimulation, he may tune out. Establish joint attention and interaction and other early learning skills to facilitate language learning. The use of sign and written words are also important as input strategies due to the strength of the visual channel in comparison to the auditory channel.

Vocabulary

Vocabulary is a relative strength for children with Down syndrome, although it grows more slowly than in the typically-developing population. Over time, there can be increasing gaps. Strategies for teaching vocabulary are listed below.

1. Use salient vocabulary that is important to the child.

2. Use specific and consistent labels (words and signs) for people, objects, and activities so the child learns to associate them.

3. Talk about and label things within the child's immediate environment as they occur and are the focus of joint attention.

4. Present and label an object; then have the child experience it by exploring it or doing an activity with it.

5. Present multiple examples of a vocabulary item, beginning with real objects, actions, and people (e.g., when teaching "ball," use balls of different colors and sizes); expand to pictures and photos.

6. Use a wide range of experiences with the item so the child can generalize, rather than memorize the concept of the item.

7. Pair labels for objects with action words (e.g., "eat cracker," "go car," "hug baby").

8. Select vocabulary to teach and model, but don't teach too many items at a time. Early vocabulary could include:

   • safety words (e.g., *no, don't, don't touch, hot, dangerous, yucky, wait, stop*)
   • people's names (e.g., the child's name, family members)
   • objects
   • actions (e.g., *go, fall, gone, up, walk, push, wash, drink, eat, night-night*)
   • body parts
   • recurrence (e.g., *more*)

9. Encourage the child to respond by following commands (e.g., finding, touching, getting, looking toward, giving) about the selected vocabulary item.

10. Use home activities and routines for selecting target vocabulary.

11. Once the child demonstrates comprehension of the label with objects, pair the object with a picture and begin the sequence again, gradually fading out the object until only the picture is used.

12. Provide repetitive practice or drill.

   • Put pictures or photos of vocabulary items in notebooks or photo albums for frequent review.
   • Build the vocabulary item into structured activities, action activities, and functional daily activities.
   • Encourage the child to identify familiar people, pictures, objects, and actions.
   • Use picture books with vocabulary themes (e.g., books about foods, animals, actions, shapes).
   • Incorporate vocabulary into novel commands or more complex ones.

13. When teaching object names, teach function and attributes along with the object. Have the child explore the item, then use it in functional tasks and with different actions.

14. When teaching actions, use different objects, places, and people associated with the actions.

   • Label the child's actions as he plays, then help the child perform actions as you label them.
   • Help the child learn the functional use of objects by using the object as the label is presented. Practice these activities in daily routines where applicable.
   • Do different actions with toys so the child doesn't memorize one function per object.
   • Have the child follow familiar action commands with objects, then introduce novel ones.

15. When teaching people's names, initially do it when the person is present, then expand to photos. Teach early pronouns (e.g., *me, mine, you, your*).

16. When teaching body parts, begin with those the child can see on himself (use a mirror). Have the child find body parts on you, himself, or a doll. Use

the body parts in functional activities (e.g., wash hands, put shoes on feet, blow nose). Then use novel activities and commands with the body parts (e.g., put earrings on ears, lipstick on mouth, lotion on legs).

17. When teaching facial expressions and emotion words, use a mirror. Imitate and label the child's facial expressions and mood states (e.g., mad, scared). Have the child imitate your facial expressions as you label them. Talk about and have the child identify facial expressions and mood states in pictures and books.

18. For the school-aged child, select vocabulary targets from classroom units or activities; preteach the vocabulary to promote classroom success; review the vocabulary to reinforce learning in the classroom.

19. Incorporate target vocabulary into language experience activities such as simple crafts, cooking, art projects, games, or routines.

20. Make photo albums, draw pictures, or create simple stories or scripts about the activities using the vocabulary. Review frequently to reinforce learning.

Associations/Categorizations

Increase the child's receptive language and preacademic skills by:

- teaching the association between objects (e.g., sock-shoe, spoon-bowl)
- teaching associations between objects/pictures and sounds (e.g., matching animal sounds to animals; matching environmental sounds to their sources)
- modeling and then having the child put together or match things that go together; begin with real objects and expand to pictures
- teaching the child how to group objects by category and naming the categories (e.g., put clothes in a dresser, food in a refrigerator, or toys in the toy box; sort objects into appropriate groups such as animals, food, or clothes)
- helping the child match objects to pictures
- having the child match and sort at a higher level (e.g., by color, by object, by shape, by function, by similarity, by category)

Following Directions

Strategies to teach the child to follow directions of increasing length and complexity include the following.

1. Gain the child's attention before giving directions.

2. Use error-free learning, particularly at the beginning.

3. Have the child reauditorize, or repeat the direction.

4. Begin with commands for behaviors that are already in the child's repertoire.

5. Follow a developmental sequence for teaching directions to gradually increase complexity. Teach:

   - safety words and directions
   - simple commands that are functional in realistic, meaningful situations (e.g., "Close door, Get the ___, Put in garbage, Pick up, Give me the ___, Go to the ___, Put away")
   - commands related to object use, toys, and people
   - commands using familiar vocabulary in daily activities and routines
   - novel commands with familiar vocabulary
   - familiar commands with new vocabulary
   - novel commands with new vocabulary
   - descriptive features by adding to the commands (e.g., "Find the large, red ball.")
   - academic, school-based directions
   - work-based directions

6. Gradually increase the length of the directions.

   - one step
   - one step with two objects
   - two-step related, simple and functional
   - two-step related, novel
   - two-step unrelated
   - three-step

Concepts

Teach functional and developmentally-appropriate concepts, providing multiple examples and experiences with the concepts.

1. Use direct teaching and repetitive practice.

2. Use the child's body and real objects to experience the concept (e.g., when teaching the word *under*, have the child get under a table, under the covers, under the bed, etc.).

3. Use daily experiences and activities (e.g., "food goes ON your plate").

4. Introduce an object with exaggerated features for teaching descriptives or one location for spatial concepts. Then have the child experience the concept using multiple examples (e.g., when teaching the concept "big," begin with one item that is obviously big; then use many items that are big such as a ball, a chair, a tree, a dog, etc.).

5. Use error-free learning by modeling, cueing, and prompting.

6. Introduce two items that are exactly the same except for the target concept (e.g., big and little ball).

   - Model the target concept "big," and use the big ball in play/functional activities. Always label the concept.
   - Prompt the child to select the big ball of the two items.
   - Give the child whatever cues he needs to be successful, including physical guidance or putting the big ball closer to him.
   - Alternate where the correct item is so the child doesn't learn to select by placement rather than by concept.
   - Use a verbal prompt (e.g., "give, get, find, show, touch, where is ___") or ask for action (e.g., "roll the big ball").
   - After the child can correctly select the big item in a set of two, expand to new item sets (e.g., hats, socks).
   - Control variables in the examples.

7. Use the *Sequence of Direction Following*, page 75 to have the child follow simple commands with the concept, then more complex or novel ones.

8. Introduce a second concept and follow the same teaching sequence.

9. Intersperse simple commands with the two concepts.

10. Teach only one of a paired concept/opposite at a time (e.g., *big/little*).

11. Teach the concept of "same/not same;" later expand this to "same/different." (These are important terms for learning concepts.)

12. Teach concepts across situations and contexts with different objects, people, and locations so the child learns the concept and doesn't memorize a command or position.

13. Help the child generalize the target concept by providing many experiences with it once he's learned the basic concept.

14. Teach the child to process and discriminate varied concept commands.

15. Teach preacademic and academic concepts (e.g., math concepts, quantity concepts).

Expressive Language and Early Speech Skill Strategies

Children with Down syndrome typically have delayed expressive language and speech skills and are late in the use of first words. They need specific, direct intervention to develop expressive communication skills.

It is important to use a Total Communication approach, incorporating verbalizations/words and gestures/signs. Signs provide a transition to speech, increase the child's ability to comprehend through his stronger visual sense, allow him to practice skills, and give him an immediate and effective way to communicate.

Sounds to First Words

The use of vocalizations, verbalizations, and true words tend to overlap so that the child may still be babbling when he begins to use some meaningful syllables and words. It is important to facilitate production of sounds and sound sequences and shape them into meaningful words.

Children build their vocabulary using words that have certain sounds and syllables, ones they can produce easily. They tend to avoid productions that are difficult for them and they are selective in the words they'll attempt. Because lexical development and phonological development mutually affect each other, it is important to work on speech early.

Strategies to facilitate early expressive communications:

1. Respond to the child's cries, sounds, and communications consistently so that he learns the power of language.

2. Give the child a reason to communicate by engineering the environment. Do not respond too quickly or anticipate the child's wants and needs as this can lead to passivity and learned helplessness.

3. Develop turn-taking and imitative skills for verbalization and signing.

4. Give the child time to initiate and respond.

5. Use repetitive practice to enhance learning.

6. Use verbal and physical cues and prompts as needed, including looking and waiting expectantly for a response.

7. Use favorite objects, people, actions, and places for first word productions.

8. Encourage the child to make sounds. (See Chapter 8, pages 88–90 for additional strategies.)

   - use movement to elicit sounds and verbalization
   - imitate the child's sounds and sound sequences; wait while looking expectantly to see if he will repeat it
   - when the child imitates it back, imitate his sound again and then add a new one
   - introduce new non-speech and speech sounds for the child to imitate

   - facilitate the use of a variety of sounds to prepare the child for word productions
   - expand vocalizations into babbling
   - extend a babbling sequence by making a change in it
   - encourage the child to make vowel sequences, consonant-vowel, and vowel-consonant syllables
   - reinforce vocalizations and verbalizations

9. Encourage the use of sounds and gestures that have communicative meaning.

   - assign communicative meaning to the child's sounds and gestures (e.g., the child says, "da," you say, "Daddy" and point to Daddy; the child puts his arms up and you say, "You want up? Up?")
   - shape vocalizations and verbalizations into meaningful communications
   - pair sounds with meaningful play and action sequences to help the child form associations. Pair specific sounds with specific activities (e.g., "whee" with swinging, "choo-choo" with train, "mmm" with yummy/tastes good)
   - pair sounds with environmental objects and animals
   - introduce new sounds and gestures. Model the target sound or gesture several times and have the child imitate.
   - teach the child to make choices using gestures, sounds or syllables
   - teach the child to identify and request objects, people, and actions using sounds and gestures
   - when child can say a sound or use a gesture to represent an object or action, encourage him to use it to request
   - accept gestures along with verbalizations as meaningful communication
   - interrupt an activity and prompt the child to use or imitate a sound or gesture to continue
   - practice sound and gesture productions throughout the day, particularly during play and in daily activities
   - use meaningful rewards for communicative attempts (e.g., give the child the requested item, perform the requested action)

- use the sounds and syllables or gestures the child can produce in real or play situations to help him generalize their use

10. Encourage the use of words or signs with the above techniques plus the following:

   - pair expressive with receptive language teaching
   - when the child requests by looking at or gesturing toward an object, label it and have him repeat using a word or sign
   - model the target sign or word and expect a response
   - use words and signs with simple motoric productions (e.g., words that use early developing consonant sounds such as bilabial sounds in "up" and "Mama")
   - work on words and signs that give the child a way to communicate with the important people around him
   - start with sound patterns that have associated social meanings (e.g., "Bye-bye, Hi, up, Mama, ba-ba" [bottle])
   - teach different types of words to prepare for syntax including action, objects, people, descriptive, location, negation, and social words
   - teach that one word/sign can be used for multiple functions (e.g., "Mama" can mean "Mama, come here", "There's Mama," or "Where's Mama?")
   - teach the child to make verbal/signed choices using "yes-no" responses or naming the desired object or activity
   - model, prompt, and shape responses
   - give the child the object or engage in the activity when he requests it
   - validate by repeating the child's communication or by responding to his meaning. Repetition and responsiveness are important.
   - accept and reinforce verbal approximations
   - use verbal and physical cueing hierarchies as needed to address imitative deficits, avoidance behaviors, and initiation difficulty. (See Chapter 3, page 29.)
   - if the child doesn't respond, give him a choice (e.g., "Is it a ___ or a ___?," "It's a ____."); name it if the child doesn't or use a question (e.g., "Is it a ____?," "No, it's a ____.")
   - ask meaningful and functional questions

- as the child begins using words/signs with less cueing and prompting, begin sabotaging the communication by stalling, misunderstanding, pausing, and waiting
- use peer modeling
- teach songs, nursery rhymes, and fingerplays

11. Teach new words following the same sequence as above plus the following:

   - read to the child, talk about what he's doing, describe and explain events and objects using short phrases or sentences
   - make scrapbooks or photo books with vocabulary themes (e.g., pets, my family, places I go, things I can do, things I like, things I eat); use pictures and written words (written captions below the pictures to name or describe the picture) for repetitive practice and review
   - make a personal dictionary containing pictures and written words of expressive targets
   - put written labels around the house to practice familiar vocabulary

Two-Word Utterances

Children with Down syndrome often have difficulty sequencing words to express ideas. They typically don't begin to use two-word utterances until they are three to four years old.

Teach the following early phrase types with words, signs, or a combination:

   agent + action ("boy go")
   action + object ("throw ball")
   agent + object ("Daddy car")
   more + object or action ("more cookie")
   nonexistence/rejection/denial ("no cookie")
   greeting ("Hi Daddy")
   possessive ("Mommy shoe")
   location ("there ball")
   descriptive ("big ball")
   temporal (now, later, "go now")
   quantitative ("two cookie")*
   conjunctive ("shoe sock")**

*   Children typically don't use morphological endings at this level, hence "two cookie" rather than "two cookies."
** Conjunctions link two items, but leave out the word *and*.

1. Begin early to move the child into verbal or signed two-word utterances using vocabulary words already in his repertoire.

2. Teach what's developmentally appropriate for the child's level and what is truly functional for him.

3. Words like *want* and *more* are important to introduce in two-word phrases to teach the child how to get his needs met.

4. Model, then prompt a response using a hierarchy of cues, including visual and multisensory input.

5. Use imitation with expansion (e.g., the child says, "Daddy car" and Mom replies, "Daddy is in the car.").

6. Respond to the child's meaning, then rephrase, restate, and provide a correct model as needed.

7. Drill and practice new skills, then use in carrier phrases and scripts.

8. Increase use and generalization by practicing new skills in natural settings.

9. Engineer the environment so the child has to use two-word phrases to make his wants, needs, and meanings known.

10. Use photo picture books to practice target two-word phrases over and over (e.g., "my mom, Daddy car, go store, puppy sleep, Cole eat").

Expanded Utterances

Children first learn word order (subject + verb + object) then they begin using morphologic word endings at the three- to four-word utterance level. As children with Down syndrome move to longer utterances, they tend to use correct word order, but have difficulty making long or complex sentences. They have difficulty with sequential processing, verbal memory, and short-term memory, all of which can affect the ability to combine words into sentences.

The use of longer sentences and syntax and morphology development are also affected by poor motor planning and poor breath control for speech and difficulty with comprehension of grammatical structures.

When teaching three-word utterances, use the same vocabulary and phrase types as for two-word utterances, but expand them by one word. Then begin increasing the length of the utterance and adding smaller parts of speech. Use the above techniques plus the following:

1. Teach three-word phrase types using words, signs, or both. Teach receptively, then practice expressively.

   - agent + action + object
   - agent + action + locative
   - action + object + locative
   - phrases with prepositions
   - phrases with modifiers
   - carrier phrases

2. Work on breath support for speech and sustained utterances.

   - sustained blowing activities (page 114)
   - strengthen abdominal muscles
   - normalize muscle tone
   - use appropriate positioning (page 106)
   - use movement activities

3. Match actions and communications to the child's level, then expand and extend them.

4. Phrase utterances in more than one way so the child learns the language rules rather than memorizing statements (e.g., when teaching the child how to use phrases with modifiers: "Misha is big. A big dog. She's a big dog.").

5. Give the child time to respond after expansions and extensions.

6. Give the child a reason to communicate using longer utterances by sabotaging the environment or misunderstanding the communication.

7. Drill and practice new skills in carrier phrases and scripts.

8. Use photo picture books to practice target phrases repeatedly:

   - add phrases to describe the pictures
   - make a "dictionary" for the classroom that includes salient school phrases and sentences. Use pictures for the non-reading child.
   - include photos of the child doing different activities and going different places
   - make a school or home diary with pictures and phrases of what the child did that day or week
   - make a "My Friends" book with pictures about friends/classmates (e.g., John is funny, Tom wears glasses.)

9. Include work on prosody to increase intelligibility in connected utterances. (See Chapter 8, page 105.)

10. Teach carrier phrases and then practice them as a part of play or in a scripted or routine activity.

11. Role-play, use barrier games or storyboards, or practice scripts of common situations.

12. Integrate into ongoing activities.

Morphology

Begin teaching morphological endings as the child reaches a three-word utterance stage. Follow a developmental progression when selecting goals.

Early morphologic endings are present progressive (*-ing*) and plurals (*-s*). These are followed by irregular past tense, possessives, regular past tense, third person singular, uncontracted copula, articles, and contracted auxiliaries.

Individuals with Down syndrome tend to have difficulty with verb tenses, question forms, pronouns, negative constructions, noun/pronoun and verb agreement, articles, conjunctions, auxiliaries, active vs. passive constructions, and subordinate clauses. (See *Two-Word Utterances*, pages 70–71 and *Expanded Utterances*, pages 71–72 for additional strategies.)

Strategies for teaching morphology include the following:

1. Model multiple examples of the structure.

2. Use real objects, actions, or people to teach structures initially, then expand to pictures and stories.

3. Model, cue, and prompt a response.

4. Rephrase, restate, and provide a correct model as needed.

5. Use signs or signals to teach and cue morphological structures (e.g., use the finger spelling for "s" for plurals and possessives).

6. Use graphic symbols to teach and cue the use of structures (e.g., when teaching the use of plurals, write the word and underline the ending "s;" point to it as the child says the word).

7. Repeatedly practice/drill new structures.

8. Use pictures or pattern books that have repeated examples of the language structure.

9. Use sentence completion, fill-in-the-blank statements, or choices for practice.

10. Role-play, use barrier games or storyboards, or practice scripts of common situations.

Augmentative Communication Strategies

Augmentative communication is often used with the child with Down syndrome to improve his language learning and use. Because of his relative strengths with visual and gestural skills, the use of gestures, signs, pictures, written word, computers, and other devices are often extremely helpful. Signing is an important expressive communication tool to augment speech.

Children with Down syndrome often can be most successful using a Total Communication approach which uses a combination of systems. (See Chapter 9, pages 119–125 for additional information.)

Pragmatic Strategies

Pragmatic skills are critical in the ability to interact with others and in the ability to make conversation and to understand others. Pragmatic skills are learned through interaction and experience. See *Early Communication Strategies*, pages 61–64 for information on early pragmatic skills.

Pragmatics and First Words

Strategies for facilitating pragmatic skills include the following:

1. Teach the child to use words or signs for early pragmatic functions, including those to:

   • protest/reject/negate
   • request objects, actions, information, recurrence
   • greet
   • call
   • offer
   • seek attention
   • comment on actions or objects
   • question
   • answer and respond

2. Teach through real-life situations, social and familiar routines, joint play activities, role-playing, and stories.

3. Get the child's attention, teaching him to maintain attention as well as eye contact.

4. Teach the child to make explicit wants and needs known.

5. Set up situations by engineering the environment so the child has to use various pragmatic functions.

6. Use enticing objects and toys with interesting actions that the child may not be able to activate by himself.

7. Use gestures and signs to support and reinforce communication.

8. Teach salient words for interactions and the language to support pragmatics.

9. Give a lot of practice (i.e., model and teach how to use new skills in everyday activities).

10. Give the child an opportunity to initiate and respond so he learns about the give-and-take of communication.

11. Teach intent by commenting on and responding to the child's verbal and nonverbal intent (e.g., The child reaches for his bottle. Mom says, "You want *bottle*? Here's *bottle*." Mom gives the bottle to the child.).

12. Teach requesting by engineering the environment (e.g., stop a desired activity, give only a small portion of a desired treat, or "forget" to put favorite toys in the tub during bath time).

13. Teach turn-taking and listening without interrupting.

Conversational Behavior/Discourse

Early pragmatics are a relative strength, but after early childhood, individuals with Down syndrome demonstrate difficulty with conversational skills. The later pragmatic and discourse skills are more difficult because the individual often doesn't have the language, processing, cognitive, and speech skills to support them. Adolescents and adults often have difficulty being understood by their conversational partners due to poor intelligibility and a lack of repair strategies necessary for communication to continue. Behaviors that can lead to communication breakdowns include difficulty with:

• attention, maintaining attention, and eye contact
• comprehension and memory skills
• interaction and turn-taking in a conversation to keep it going
• responding to language (Note: Individuals with Down syndrome often take longer to respond, have difficulty formulating a response, and may miss the communication turn or moment.)
• initiating a conversation, opening and closing a conversation
• choosing a topic and maintaining a topic
• asking conversational questions
• taking the listener's knowledge and perspective into account

- giving related answers
- making conversational repairs such as clarifying or correcting, adding additional information, or requesting clarification
- knowing when to pause, how to interrupt, how to provide feedback to the listener, and the proper physical distance to maintain between the speaker and listener
- reading the facial expressions and emotions of others
- regulating the behavior of others
- describing, predicting, hypothesizing, giving reasons, and instructing
- understanding sarcasm, slang, humor, and idioms

The emphasis in intervention should be on developing the child's ability to understand and use communication effectively. Teach the child how to initiate a conversation, maintain a conversation, and make conversational repairs. Teach higher-level discourse skills for those who are at that level. Read Greenspan (1998) for ideas for setting up interactions and expanding verbal exchanges. To facilitate conversational behavior and discourse:

- Teach salient words and expressions (e.g., slang, social words and phrases like "How're you doing?", and greetings).
- Teach proxemics (e.g., the distance to stand from other person, shaking hands, greeting rather than hugging).
- Teach the child how to interpret facial expressions, mood states, and social cues.
- Teach the child conversational repair strategies and give him time to repair his own messages (e.g., repeating, rewording, providing more information, slowing the rate, using appropriate stress and separation of syllables and words, and using signs or Total Communication).
- Teach the child how to recognize conversational breakdowns or misunderstandings.
- Teach the child how to ask for more information or to clear up a misunderstanding for clarification.
- Teach the child how to use recasts to rephrase content that's misunderstood.
- Prompt the child to stay on topic by telling him, "We're talking about (subject)."
- Use role playing to practice pragmatic skills during various scenarios.

- Teach conversational/topic maintenance.
- Teach the child to take the listener's knowledge and perspective into account.
  - ▶ use pictures that vary in one aspect (Receptively, have the child find the one you describe. Expressively, have the child describe the picture or differences between the pictures.)
  - ▶ use barrier games or draw pictures while following directions where the child alternates between the listener role and speaker role
- Use a story in cartoon form and have the child tell the story to another who cannot see the picture.
- Have the child describe a movie, retell a story or event, or describe how a toy works.
- Teach comprehension and use of synonyms, antonyms, homonyms, inferences, idioms, metaphors, and abstractions.

Auditory/Language Processing Strategies

Therapy should address selective attention, vigilance, memory and sequential memory, discrimination, association, synthesis and analysis skills, and word-retrieval skills. Strategies to increase auditory and language processing follow.

1. Get the child's attention first. Use movement activities and sensory stimulation in the activity to help build alertness and focus. Cue the child to watch and listen.

2. Encourage the child to listen to the entire instruction, direction, or question before beginning a response.

3. Encourage task completion.

4. Teach that every activity has a sequence with a beginning and end.

5. Pair the weaker learning modality with the stronger one and teach through the stronger one (e.g., Pair the weaker auditory system with visual input and cues through the use of multisensory cues, signing, and written word).

6. Give the child time to process. Give him time to organize and formulate a response, but also help reduce his latency before responding by cueing him to respond.

7. Use a hierarchy of cueing. (See Chapter 3, page 29.)

8. Use auditory trainers, FM systems, or hearing aids to supplement hearing and auditory processing as needed.

9. Begin with short, structured tasks with no distracters and error-free learning. Gradually add distracters and increased complexity of tasks.

10. Begin with familiar vocabulary, commands, and concepts and expand to novel ones.

11. Reinforce the child's attempts; provide the level of reinforcement needed to keep the child on task.

12. Improve the ability to follow directions that gradually increase in complexity; use in structured settings with drill, modeling, and cueing and then expand to real-life situations.

   - use vocabulary and concepts in the child's repertoire
   - build up to longer and novel directions
   - use real-life situations, recipes, household tasks, and craft projects
   - use prompts and cues, including visual cues such as using pointing, pictures, gestures, and signs

---

Sequence of Direction Following

- one-step functional directions
- one-step directions with target vocabulary and concepts
- one-step more abstract directions
- two-step related directions
- two-step unrelated directions
- three-step directions
- novel directions
- following longer, more complex directions
- directions with elements embedded
- following directions in sequential order

---

13. Increase memory and retrieval skills.

   - Use a cueing hierarchy, beginning with maximum cueing and gradually reducing the level of cueing and support.
   - Reauditorize or rehearse (i.e., repeat information to be remembered).
   - Chunk information (i.e., group information that goes together).
   - Make associations to cue memory.
   - Use imagery (i.e., visualize what needs to be remembered).
   - Teach the adolescent or adult to make lists and check them, and/or to use a daily planner or calendar.
   - Practice following directions in sequence beginning with two-step directions; cue the child to perform them in the order of presentation.

14. Increase auditory association skills.

   - Pair animals and the sounds they make.
   - Pair environmental objects and the sounds they make.
   - Do fingerplays with associated songs.
   - Match objects or pictures to sounds associated with them.
   - Match objects or pictures to spoken words.
   - Introduce sound-symbol association matching letters and sounds.

15. Increase auditory discrimination skills.

   - Match animal, environment, or instrument sounds to objects or pictures.
   - Match voices to people or their pictures.
   - Match pairs of words or determine if the words sound the same or different.
   - Discriminate sound features (e.g., *loud/soft, same/different*).

16. Increase synthesis (i.e., putting parts together to form a whole) and analysis (i.e., breaking a whole into its parts) skills.

   - Use pictures paired with segmented words or words with a syllable or ending omitted; show the child how to match the picture to the spoken word.

- Repeat the above, but use two pictures so the child must actively listen and process. Gradually increase the number of pictures or written words available.
- Extend to spoken tasks with no pictures.
- Use learning experiences or activities such as crafts, cooking, or art, and ask questions that lead the child to talk about parts of the experiences and to make conclusions.

Question Use and Response Strategies

Adults tend to use questions as a primary communication tool with children with Down syndrome because the children often fail to initiate and respond. Questions can be effective when they are used to get attention, to elicit responses, to gauge what the child knows, to teach turn-taking, and to elicit responses. However, questions can become ineffective or encourage the child to be a passive conversational partner if they are used too frequently or as the primary pattern for interacting with the child.

The child needs to learn how to use questions appropriately to gain knowledge and to enter and continue conversations. Questions should be taught receptively, expressively, and pragmatically. Strategies for developing comprehension and use of questions follow.

1. Use questions carefully. Use those that are functional, useful, and keep a conversation going.

2. Teach listening behavior (e.g., to watch and listen, to make eye contact, and to wait for the whole question before responding).

3. Use questions in the context of daily activities.

4. Model questions and responses; prompt as needed.

5. Ask questions the child is capable of responding to and give him practice responding to mastered question forms.

6. Use structured tasks to teach how to use and respond to questions as well as incorporating them into daily activities and play; then practice asking and answering questions.

7. Role-play different scenarios and daily activities and use scripts (e.g., practice going to a store and asking for a specific item, getting directions from someone, or making conversation with a friend).

8. Practice the use of questions and answers in the community in community-based instruction (e.g., on a field trip to the bakery, the child may use questions such as "Do you have chocolate donuts? How much do they cost?").

9. Wait before repeating, rephrasing, restating, or answering a question.

10. Use books and reading activities that provide visual support.

11. Make picture/photo books that target specific questions forms (e.g., a "who" book with pictures of salient people, a "where" book that has pictures of favorite or common places).

12. Teach and practice one question form at a time; gradually incorporate a second question form.

13. Begin with simple questions (e.g., *yes/no, what, who, where*).

14. Teach the child how to use questions to gain more information and to clarify.

15. Teach the social use of questions (e.g., "How are you?" "What's your name?").

16. Teach the child how to use questions and answers for problem solving and give him experience in doing this.

17. Engineer the environment to encourage the use of questions.

Higher Language/Abstract Language Skill Strategies

Higher language skills typically are difficult for individuals with Down syndrome because of their cognitive limitations and the abstract nature of higher language skills. With training and appropriate and continued intervention, some individuals with Down syndrome can learn to comprehend and use higher language skills. All of the following higher language skills can be areas of intervention for individuals with Down syndrome.

Higher Language Skills

- explaining, describing, retelling, reordering, thinking skills
- similarities/differences
- similes/analogies
- homonyms/antonyms
- categorizing and subcategorizing
- problem solving
- *if-then* and *why-because* statements
- multiple-meaning words
- analysis and synthesis skills
- idioms, figures of speech, and slang
- academic language including community-based language

To teach higher language skills:

1. Model examples of higher language structures.

2. Teach in structured contexts and provide repeated practice, initially using error-free learning.

3. Use pictures, drawings, or written words to illustrate and reinforce learning.

4. Make books with examples of structures such as idioms, *why-because* statements, and similes. Have the child generate phrases or sentences using the terms and write them in the book.

5. Use barrier games, scripted activities, and learning experiences.

6. Use routines and activities to teach and to practice.

7. Practice the structures in controlled situations, new situations, and then in the community.

8. Use new examples of the structures and/or use the structures in different settings with different people.

9. When developing specific objectives and goals, consult with parents, teachers, job coaches, employers, and community contacts.

10. Teach language important for academics and work:

    - use the curriculum and textbooks for selection of vocabulary and concepts
    - preteach vocabulary and concepts, particularly those with multiple meanings
    - teach reasoning and thinking skills
    - use hands-on, experiential teaching
    - use multisensory cues

Functional Life Skill Strategies for Teens and Adults

Language therapy should continue through late adolescence or early adulthood and should focus on the use of complex sentences, morpheme use, speech intelligibility, functional or higher language skills, and pragmatic skills. During adulthood, the individual should be monitored for Alzheimer's and dementia.

1. Teach developmentally-appropriate social, interaction, and language skills.

2. Teach current vocabulary (e.g., slang, idioms) that facilitates conversational skills and peer interaction.

3. Develop augmentative communication systems as needed to help communicate in life settings.

4. Teach specific tasks and language necessary for work settings (e.g., teach the steps for preparing the salad bar at a restaurant along with questions the individual may need to ask like "Where are the tomatoes?") as well as constructive work-related habits (e.g., personal hygiene, being on time).

5. Teach language necessary for community settings by practicing various scenarios (e.g., buying clothes).

6. Increase planning and problem-solving skills.

7. Increase the ability to recognize and make conversational repairs.

8. Repeatedly practice skills, then use role playing and scripts, and practice in actual settings.

9. Teach organizational and memory strategies such as reauditorization and rehearsal. Use notebooks with pictures to help remember how to manage daily activities and routines (e.g., catching the bus, using the phone, doing laundry).

10. Teach the adolescent or adult how to navigate through his environment at home, at school, in the community, on the job, during leisure activities, and socially.

Functional Daily Living Skills

- make change, count money, pay bills, budget
- make a grocery list, use coupons
- make purchases at a store
- plan a menu, follow a simple recipe
- shop (e.g., understand ads and signs in a store, size tags in clothing, departments in a store)
- take/leave a message
- comprehend safety and information words
- understand labels (e.g., poison, washable vs. nonwashable, edible vs. nonedible, precautions, medicine labels)
- get and use directions
- manage public transportation
- comprehend the meaning of signs and messages (e.g., Detour, Exit)
- complete a job interview or answer questions on an application
- follow work directions in sequence
- complete assigned tasks
- follow directions to get to and from salient places
- order at a restaurant
- buy tickets for a movie or concert

Chapter 8: Speech Development and Intervention

General Information about Down Syndrome Speech

Speech intelligibility in children with Down syndrome is affected by anatomical and physiological differences as well as delayed or disordered phonological development. It can also be affected by:

- hearing loss and recurrent ear infections
- low tone
- reduced muscle strength
- impaired respiration/phonation
- problems in planning and/or implementing the sequence of sounds necessary for speech
- difficulty with coarticulatory movements
- distortion in the way sensory information is organized and interpreted
- prosody disturbances
- voice and resonance disturbances
- disfluency
- difficulty processing information (particularly through the auditory channel)

Anatomical and physiological differences have an impact on all aspects of the production of speech sounds and connected speech (i.e., respiration, phonation, articulation, resonance, motor planning and sequencing, fluency, and voice).

1. Skeletal abnormalities of the mouth and skull can result in a habitual open-mouth posture.

   - high narrow palate with decreased volume of the oral cavity (i.e., a small mouth)
   - malocclusion due to underdevelopment of the maxilla and/or protrusion of the mandible with abnormally-shaped and/or missing teeth
   - underdevelopment of the frontal and paranasal sinuses and nasal passages and recurrent upper respiratory infections
   - poorly developed facial skeleton diminishes the ability of the muscles to close the jaw

2. Differences in brain development can affect motor-speech coordination and the ability to process information.

3. Lax joints affect jaw stability and the ability to grade jaw openings.

4. Overall hypotonia throughout the body affects muscle strength, precision, and coordinated movements of the speech mechanism. The low muscle tone can affect respiration/phonation, velopharyngeal closure, and vocal fold seals. This difficulty with respiration/phonation and valving at the vocal folds and velopharyngeal mechanism results in a reduced ability to produce connected speech and also in resonance and voice problems.

5. Poor postural tone leads to poor positioning of the body. The back typically is slumped with the head back toward the shoulders. This leads to poor respiration/phonation (i.e., the coordination of the respiratory mechanism and the vocal fold functioning involving starting, stopping, and grading airflow) and an open-mouth position with a protruding tongue.

6. Reduced muscle strength and tone contributes to a habitual pattern of a slack, open jaw with a protrusive tongue position.

   - Approximately 1/2 to 3/4 of the individuals with Down syndrome have an enlarged tongue. However, the tongue may be normal in size, but look large because of the small oral cavity and the low tone in the tongue.
   - Low tone in the tongue results in difficulty with central grooving, tension, retraction, or elevation of the tongue. This causes a general front-back movement pattern rather than precise articulatory movements.
   - A tongue thrust/swallowing pattern is present with the tongue moving forward during swallowing rather than using a mature tongue pattern.
   - There is a tendency toward enlarged tonsils and adenoids which encourage the tongue-forward positioning so the child can breathe.
   - Positioning the tongue in protrusion can become a habit. The sensory stimulation experienced when the tongue is protruded may reinforce this position.

Speech Patterns
Patterns often seen in the speech of children with Down syndrome include the following:

1. A Pattern of Phonological Processes

   These processes are the sound simplifications or substitution patterns that young children use to make speech productions easier. They include processes such as final consonant deletion, substitutions, and cluster reduction.

   The child with Down syndrome generally uses these processes much longer than her typically-developing

peers. Most typically-developing children don't use these past the age of five.

Phonological simplification is the primary pattern seen in children with Down syndrome. The most common processes are final consonant deletion and cluster reduction followed by simplification of nasals and liquids. Other common patterns include a high percentage of errors on stop consonants and a fronting or backing pattern.

The least common errors occur with syllable deletion and reduplication (i.e., repeating a syllable in a word), although there is a pattern of weak syllable deletion (e.g., "ehphant" for "elephant").

The phonemes that have the highest percentages of error are /s/ (the most impaired phoneme), /d, t, n/ (these often are omitted, particularly in the medial and final position of words), /r, z, l, s/ and /r/ blends. For older children, there are persistent errors on /s, sh, ch, j/.

2. Dysarthria

   Because of neurological differences and hypotonia, children with Down syndrome often show evidence of dysarthria, a neurologically-based speech disorder resulting in difficulty with control and coordination of the complex movements needed for speech.

   There may be disturbances in the strength, speed, coordination, precision, tone, and range of movement of the articulators.

   Dysarthria results in overall difficulties producing speech, rather than difficulty producing individual speech sounds. Speech errors tend to be consistent in nature.

3. Apraxia of Speech

   Children with Down syndrome can have speech motor planning and control problems which result in difficulty producing and sequencing the volitional movements needed for speech. Speech articulation, coordination, timing, and rate may all be affected.

Difficulty processing sequential information underlies the oral-motor planning/control difficulty. Also, distortion in the way sensory information is organized and interpreted may interfere with development of skilled oral-motor patterns of movement.

Children with apraxia of speech exhibit difficulty with syllable structure control. The child may be inefficient in sequencing and blending sounds into syllables or words and longer utterances. As the production and sequencing demands increase, the child has more difficulty with speech intelligibility.

This is a motor programming problem, not a muscular one, so sound errors tend to be inconsistent and can be dependent on the length and complexity of the speech message.

4. Auditory Processing

Children with Down syndrome tend to have difficulty remembering ordered information presented auditorily. They may have problems with sequential processing which affects speech intelligibility.

5. Other Factors Affecting Speech Production or Intelligibility

Development of meaningful speech takes a long time for children with Down syndrome. Many don't consistently use conventional words before the age of three years. This results in a lack of speech practice in comparison to their typically-developing peers. The speech delay is correlated to the delays in motor development and motor-planning. Delays in imitative verbal and gestural abilities may also contribute to the slow pace of development of meaningful speech. The child with Down syndrome may also have poor awareness of speech errors.

Sixty to 80% of children with Down syndrome have hearing deficits. Twenty to 50% have recurring otitis media.

Children with Down syndrome have greater visual skills than auditory skills. They learn better by watching and doing, rather than through listening.

There may be a low motivation to communicate which is a result of repeated failure or difficulty with verbal imitation and production. They avoid words they can't produce and are selective in the words they'll attempt. This results in limited attempts at speech sounds and words. Speech avoidance can also result in delay of emergence of two-word utterances and limit the selection of words to be combined.

Prosody disturbances (i.e., the melody of speech) can affect overall speech intelligibility.

- the rate tends to be fast, with the child speaking rapidly or in spurts
- restricted intonational contours (e.g., not using rising inflection for questions)
- rhythm or timing problems
- lack of separation between syllables and words
- equalization of syllable and word stress

Children with Down syndrome may talk quietly. Their soft volume can result from hearing loss and low tone which affects breath support for loudness.

Some adolescents and adults with Down syndrome may be disfluent, particularly those who are more verbal.

Many children with Down syndrome have a breathy, husky voice or hoarse voice quality. This is secondary to low tone in the larynx, poor vocal fold seal, allergies, and/or poor breath support for speech.

Some children with Down syndrome may have difficulty with the tonal quality of their speech.

- hyponasality: due to enlarged tonsils/adenoids, allergies, and/or small nasal cavities and sinuses

- hypernasality: due to short velum, flaccid muscles, and/or difficulty with velopharyngeal closure

Intervention

Speech is a whole body process. Age-appropriate speech skills require appropriate respiration and breath support; appropriate postural tone; adequate muscle tone and strength; articulatory stability, grading, control, and movement; and appropriate vocal fold functioning. Speech can be influenced by a weakness, incoordination, or breakdown in any part of the systems.

Down syndrome impacts all of these systems. Treatment for Down syndrome speech should incorporate principles and techniques from many treatment approaches including phonology, dysarthria, apraxia of speech, and aural rehabilitation.

Movement and Positioning

Movement and positioning can help strengthen muscle tone and postural stability in the child with Down syndrome. Muscle tone is the degree of tension in the muscles at rest or during movement. The muscular system provides support for the skeletal system and allows for movement and stability. Postural tone is the ability to maintain appropriate body positions. It is dependent on appropriate muscle tone.

Stability means the co-contraction of muscles to hold the body against gravity and/or to hold the joints in place to allow movement at other joints. This stability allows for greater mobility so that movement may be precise and skilled. Stability and mobility need to be balanced for every movement.

Decreased postural and muscle tone and strength are characteristic in children with Down syndrome. Also, many children with Down syndrome need to increase their inspiration of air, extend their expiration of air, and grade their airflow to produce connected speech. Movement activities can help in these areas plus facilitate and promote alertness, organization, focus, calming, mobility, and coordination, as well as provide stability and support for the various systems involved in the speech process. Some examples of activities follow.

1. Movement patterns combining vestibular and proprioceptive inputs help in development of muscle tone, postural control, and respiratory function.

Activities could include jumping, hopping, swinging, running, bouncing, exercises, and yoga.

2. Movements which require oral resistance stimulate oral-motor proprioceptors. Activities could include resistive sucking and blowing.

Respiration/Breath Control

Respiration provides the energy for the speech system. Poor respiration/breath control may result in the use of shorter utterances, omission of word endings, syllable deletion, or inaudible speech. Techniques to improve respiration/breath control include the following:

- Use gross motor movement activities (e.g., jumping, skipping, dancing).
- Have the child lie on her stomach on the floor during speech practice. This provides some stability and input to the abdominal muscles.
- Have the child sit, stand, or lie on her back. Push in on the child's diaphragm as she produces speech.
- Have the child lie over a big ball on her stomach. Hold her at the hips and push into the ball to bounce her.
- Have the child take a deep breath as she raises her arms over her head. Then have the child blow the air out in a long, easy expiration as she lowers her arms to her sides.
- Have the child lie over a big ball or bolster on her stomach. Help her roll forward to touch her hands to the floor, then back to the starting position.
- Build abdominal strength via crunch-type sit ups, yoga, or other exercises.

Body Positioning

Body positioning is extremely important for the child with Down syndrome for feeding, oral-motor activities, and speech tasks. Appropriate body positioning can provide stability of the body which then allows for greater mobility, and skilled and precise movements.

There is a reciprocal influence between posture and the respiratory system. Stability is needed through the spine in order to gain mobility in the rib cage and for the respiratory system to develop maximum efficiency.

Positioning considerations include the child's overall posture with proper alignment of the hips, shoulder, head, and neck. Any forward or backward tilting of the pelvis in sitting or standing can influence head control, breathing, voicing, mouth control, and/or articulatory movement.

Typical postures noted in children with Down syndrome include pelvic tilting due to low tone in the trunk. This position tends to result in hyperflexion of the neck which then throws the jaw off alignment and can result in an open-mouth posture with the tongue forward. Slumped positions also result in decreased respiratory efficiency.

When seated in a chair, the child should be in 90-90-90 positioning (i.e., hips, knees, and ankles flexed at a 90 degree angle) with the back straight and the feet flat on the floor or a footrest. The child's head should be in midline with the chin slightly tucked. If the head is tilted back with the chin up or sunk back toward the shoulders, a tongue-forward position with the lips open results.

During speech practice, the child may also lie prone on her stomach, propped on her elbows that are directly under her shoulders. Her head should be forward and up, not sunk between the shoulders. This may be modified by having the child rest her chin on her cupped hands between her palms or on a fist to provide additional jaw support and stability.

Other positions include having the child sit on the floor with her legs crossed. Provide back support if needed. A young child may be seated in the therapist's lap on the floor with her back against the therapist for support. Use adaptive seating devices as needed.

Whenever the child is seated or standing, encourage a straight back. Tapping or rubbing at the base of the spine often will bring the child upright.

Oral-Motor Stimulation

Oral-motor stimulation is direct intervention to the speech mechanism through tactile and proprioceptive cues which are used to reduce abnormal oral movement patterns and to encourage more skilled movement patterns. (Proprioception is the information that arises from your own movement, the sensory information you get from your muscles and joints.)

Oral-motor facilitation involves direct touch input to the speech mechanism to achieve articulatory placement and accurate sound production. Feedback from that touch and articulatory movement is then used to help the child bring speech production under his voluntary control. (See Appendix A, pages 106-114, for more information on the following.)

1. Facilitation techniques include touch, movement, positioning, and proprioception or sensory feedback. Speech generally is monitored through auditory and proprioceptive feedback. These activities can facilitate jaw stability and grading, increased oral awareness, oral muscle tone, lip closure, tongue mobility and placement, separation of jaw and tongue function, and precise articulatory movement.

2. Begin oral-motor stimulation outside the mouth on the face and gradually work inside. Stimulation outside the mouth can help increase sensory awareness; normalize sensitivity and tone; and lead to control, strength, and precision of articulatory movement. It can also prepare the child to accept stimulation inside the mouth.

3. Make sure the child is positioned in the 90-90-90 position with her head upright in midline for oral-motor intervention. During oral-motor stimulation, the child's mouth should be open in a neutral position rather than opened widely.

4. When applying stimulation to one side of the face, jaw, gums, lips, or tongue, always do the same to the other side. Symmetrical application is important.

5. Quick touches, vibration, or stretches will increase muscle tone.

6. Generally repeat each oral-motor activity three times. Always follow oral-motor stimulation with a functional activity (e.g., eating or speech practice).

7. Never force the child to accept oral-motor stimulation until she is ready for it. Work at her pace, and gradually introduce oral-motor tasks.

8. Not all oral-motor techniques must be implemented. Choose several each session that are applicable to the particular child.

Oral Sensitivity

It is necessary to determine if the child has normal sensitivity, hypersensitivity, or hyposensitivity in the oral area. Some children are overly sensitive in the oral area, making it hard to work in the mouth. Some are undersensitive so they are not very aware of what's happening in the mouth. Normalizing oral tactile sensitivity is important in order to increase the child's ability to accept direct touch to the articulators, and to increase her awareness of the articulatory structures, their movements, and their contact points.

Determine which stimulation techniques work best with each child. Watch the child's responses for areas of weakness, lack of control, over-sensitivity to touch, and tone variations. Target these areas to normalize responses. You may need to begin with short sessions of oral-motor stimulation and gradually increase the length of stimulation over time.

Consult with a pediatric OT or PT as needed to determine which activities or stimulations may be appropriate for a particular child, particularly for children with tactile defensiveness.

When implementing touch techniques to the body, face, and mouth, generally use deep, firm pressure. This can be used for desensitization or facilitation. Some children, however may respond best to light pressure.

Wear protective gloves when doing any oral-motor activities in or around the child's mouth. Always check for latex allergies before doing any oral-motor activities.

I. Hypersensitivity

Hypersensitivity is an over-reaction to touch. It is also called tactile defensiveness. The child with Down syndrome may show some of these characteristics in different degrees including the following:

- an aversion to being touched. She may prefer to be the one who initiates touching.
- an overreaction to minor bumps and falls
- sensitivity to certain textures of clothing, or avoidance of play with certain textures like sand, glue, or finger paint
- an avoidance of certain foods because of the texture or smell, or gagging on certain foods. She may be a picky eater.
- an open-mouth posture when chewing to avoid manipulation of the food
- a strong dislike for having her face washed or wiped, for having her teeth brushed, or having her hair cut
- a tendency to be overly ticklish

The child with oral tactile defensiveness tends to reject oral-motor stimulation. In this case, begin by decreasing sensitivity away from the child's face, then gradually work toward the child's face and mouth.

a. Begin with texture experiences on the child's hands and arms such as rubbing lotion on them, wiping them with a towel, finding toys hidden in a large container of beans/sand/rice/pebbles, or finger painting with shaving cream or pudding.

b. Gradually work toward the face, beginning desensitization outside the child's mouth by wiping her face with a washcloth, rubbing it with lotion, or patting and stroking it using deep pressure.

c. Then desensitize inside the child's mouth. Introduce techniques gradually using slow movements with firm, deep pressure. Use an Infa-dent®, washcloth, or Toothette® to stroke along the upper inner gum line from molar to molar in a back and forth direction three times.

Use your gloved thumb to exert downward pressure on the midline of the child's lower jaw (i.e., hook your thumb over the lower incisors and press down) for a few seconds. Use a gloved finger to maintain pressure for three to five seconds on the midline of the child's tongue. Stroke the roof of the child's mouth from front to back, being careful not to elicit a gag reflex.

Consult a professional trained in sensory/oral defensiveness prior to implementing these techniques as needed.

d. Using food experiences can be a less intrusive method of introducing stimulation inside the mouth. Never force food experiences on the child.

Use foods that have different textures such as:

- crunchy (e.g., pretzels, crackers, carrot sticks, pickles, apples)
- chewy (e.g., raisins, Fruit Roll-Ups®, dried fruit, Gummy Bears®)
- sour (e.g., Sour Patch Kids® candy, lemon slices, cranberry juice, dill pickles)
- spicy (e.g., pepperoni slices, Hot Tamales® candy)
- sweet (e.g., candy, fruit)

2. Hyposensitivity

Hyposensitivity is a decreased awareness of touch or an under-reaction to touch. The hyposensitive child may:

- crave touch experiences (e.g., chewing on her clothes or fingers, or spending too long brushing her teeth)
- have a decreased awareness and responsivity to touch, pain, or temperature
- have a poor perception of where her tongue is in her mouth, or where the articulators are in relation to each other
- drool in the absence of teething
- have a tendency to seek foods that provide increased input (e.g., spicy, crunchy)
- have a tendency to overstuff her mouth when eating. She may be unaware that she has food in and around her mouth after eating and be a messy eater.
- have an under-reactive gag reflex

Begin working on the child's face and progress to her mouth quickly. Use deep pressure, a cloth with rough texture (e.g., washcloth), and/or cold temperature to increase awareness in the oral area.

Apply stimulation much the same way as with the hypersensitive child, but use quicker touches and spend more time in the oral area.

Use crunchy, spicy, or chewy foods to provide proprioceptive input. Chewing a wad of cinnamon gum (several sticks in the mouth at the same time) can provide proprioceptive input through heavy chewing.

Food Experiences

> **Always check for food allergies and sensitivities before giving the child any food, particularly before using peanut products.**

Appropriate food experiences can provide stimulation inside the child's mouth which is less intrusive than direct touch techniques to the articulators. Food experiences can help normalize oral sensitivity and tone, facilitate sensory awareness in the oral area, facilitate jaw stability and grading, and facilitate oral movements.

To alert the oral cavity, have the child take a few bites or chew up a food that has a sour or tingly taste (e.g., lemon, sour candy, dill pickles) or is hot (e.g., Hot Tamales® or War Heads® candy). You can also have the child chew cinnamon, spearmint, or peppermint gum.

Improve the child's jaw grading by having her bite crackers, carrot sticks, or celery sticks or chew on chewy candy or foods such as raisins or chewing gum. Have her bite and chew with her lips closed.

Improve the child's tongue function by putting a sticky food such as peanut butter, jelly, or marshmallow cream above the center of the child's upper lip, on the alveolus, or the palate. Have the child lick it off with her tongue.

Improve independent tongue function by holding a Popsicle®, spoon coated with peanut butter (or other sticky food), tongue depressor, or sucker in front of the child's mouth. Have her protrude her tongue and lick the object. Make sure the child doesn't move her head.

Be aware that sugar increases drooling. Be cautious using sugary foods for a child who continues to drool.

The Face and Lips

The muscles of the face and lips are so intrinsically related, they exhibit functional unity. You can't get fine, coordinated lip movement without cheek muscle function. Use touch and movement to facilitate face and lip muscle tone, movement, control, and sensitivity.

> Refer to Appendix A: *Illustrated Oral-Motor Techniques* at the end of this chapter (pages 106–114) for illustrations and explanations of the starred (*) techniques.

a. Normalize sensitivity and increase facial tone by applying deep pressure to the facial muscles and lips.

b. Tap or give firm pats* to the cheeks, jaw, lips, and under the chin. (page 106)

c. Rub or stroke the muscles of the face, beginning at the point of origin of each facial muscle and following it to where it inserts into or around the lips. Stroke around the lips in a circular motion. Use the fingers or a washcloth.

d. Use manual vibration* following the course of the facial muscles from the point of origin to the point of insertion at the lips. Vibrate around the lips, beginning at the center of the upper lip and moving in a circle around the lips back to the starting point. (page 107)

e. Use sustained blowing* or resistive sucking activities*. (page 114)

f. Have the child imitate isolated facial movements such as smiling or using an exaggerated pucker to throw kisses.

g. Have the child imitate sequential facial movements (e.g., alternate between a lip retraction [smile] and lip rounding [kiss]).

h. Facilitate lip strength and a variety of lip movements including lip rounding/pursing, lip closure, and retraction/spreading. (page 109) Lip rounding techniques include pucker resistance* and smile resistance*. You can also use blowing and/or resistive sucking activities*. (page 114) Lip closure techniques include the following:

- rubbing or tapping on and around the lips to increase tone and to increase sensory awareness of contact points
- manual vibration* along the facial muscles (page 107)
- resistance activities such as having the child press her lips together tightly and resist as you try to open her lips. Then put a washcloth, toy, tongue blade, straw, or food item between the child's lips and ask her to hold onto it with her lips as you gently try to pull it out. She should use only her lips, not her teeth.
- bunny nose technique* (page 108)
- V-pressure technique* (page 108)
- mustache press technique* (page 109)
- lip stroke technique* (page 109)
- sustained blowing and/or resistive sucking activities* (page 114)

The Jaw

Jaw stability and control are extremely important for the child with Down syndrome for feeding, oral-motor, and speech tasks. Jaw stability and control can be affected by postural and muscle tone in the body and face, a lax mandibular joint, and a habitual open-mouth posture.

Initially the mouth functions as a total unit (jaw, tongue, lower and upper lip). Independent, controlled movements of the tongue depend on jaw stability. Postural stability of the jaw should be achieved by 24 to 36 months in typically-developing children, but finer grading ability continues to develop over time.

Adequate control and stability of the jaw means that the jaw is positioned in the midline, there is appropriate opening and closing of the jaw with symmetrical movements, and the jaw opening is graded (increments of opening).

Techniques to facilitate jaw stability and graded movements include the following:

l. When applying oral stimulation to the jaw, make sure the child's back is straight and her head is in midline with her chin slightly tucked. Don't let the child's head move forward, backward, up, or down during the activity as this defeats the purpose of the activity.

2. Provide jaw stability by doing resistance activities. Resistance is pressure applied to muscles as the child is purposefully moving in the opposite direction.

   - Do the resistance to jaw opening technique* and the resistance to jaw closing technique*. (page 107)
   - Place a washcloth, a piece of thick licorice, or a piece of Fruit Roll-Ups® between the child's front teeth and pull on it as she keeps her teeth closed on it for jaw resistance.

3. Provide proprioceptive input by pushing inward on the point of the chin* with deep pressure for a few seconds and/or massaging the muscles around the temporomandibular joint. (page 108)

4. Tap along the mandible borders using quick taps.

5. Improve jaw grading by biting crackers, carrot sticks, celery sticks, or foods of different thickness or density.

6. Resistive sucking techniques* using different sucking strengths and different size straws and/or aquarium tubing can facilitate jaw grading. (page 114)

7. Sustained blowing activities* can facilitate jaw stability and grading. (page 114)

8. A bite block* such as a straw, thin pretzel, or coffee stirrer between the molars during speech tasks provides jaw stability. (page 108)

9. Have the child cup her chin* in both hands or place her chin on her fist to provide jaw stability as she practices speech sounds and words. (page 108)

The Tongue

Children with Down syndrome have reduced muscle tone and strength throughout the body including the tongue. This leads to difficulty with precise and controlled tongue movements during speech and a tongue thrust pattern during speech, feeding, and at rest.

Increase muscle tone and strength in the tongue by using tapping and resistance activities. Often the tongue is not too large in the child with Down syndrome, but low tone in the tongue and a small oral cavity make it look that way. Also, the jaw tends to be too mobile and unstable and the tonsils and adenoids may be enlarged, all of which encourage a forward carriage of the tongue.

- Use one finger to quickly tap from the front to the back of the tongue along the midline. Be careful not to elicit the child's gag reflex.
- Tap under the child's chin at the base of the tongue.
- Tap along the tongue front and tip.
- Press into the child's tongue tip with a finger as the child pushes back (resistance). Make sure she uses only her tongue and not her head to push.

Facilitate tongue grooving, elevation (front, tip, back and sides), retraction, and spreading of the tongue for speech sound production. Refer to *Speech Sound Groups and Specific Intervention for Each*, pages 95–104 for specific techniques to facilitate each of these tongue movements.

Facilitate separation of jaw and tongue function to develop independent movements of the tongue.

- Use jaw resistance* activities. (page 107)
- Use a bite block* during speech productions (e.g., small straw, thin tongue depressor, cocktail straw, coffee stirrer, commercial bite block). (page 108)
- Place a sticky food such as peanut butter, marshmallow cream, or jelly on the child's teeth, alveolus, or palate and have the child use her tongue to remove the food. Use a bite block to reduce jaw movements if needed.

If the child continues to exhibit abnormal oral movement patterns, it is important to figure out what is causing the problem and to intervene at that level. If the child is having difficulty with precise and coordinated tongue movements because of poor jaw stability and control, work on the jaw prior to addressing the tongue. If the poor jaw control is due to poor postural stability or muscle tone, begin work there.

Reduce a habitual tongue protrusion pattern with the following:

- Position the child with a straight back and the head upright in midline with the chin slightly tucked.
- Facilitate postural and muscle tone through movement activities. (See *Movement and Positioning*, page 82.)
- Facilitate appropriate jaw positioning and closure using jaw activities. (See *The Jaw*, pages 86–87.) Provide external support as needed by placing your thumb and finger under the mandible and the chin.
- Check for enlarged tonsils and adenoids which may encourage a tongue-forward positioning.
- Facilitate muscle tone in the face and lips by tapping or patting the cheeks and lips using quick movements with deep pressure. Stroke each lip from center to corner, briefly holding*. (page 109)
- Facilitate tongue retraction* by using tapping, stroking, and resistance techniques. Briefly pull forward on the tongue and release. Rub along the sides of the tongue from the middle to the back of the tongue. Manually elevate the tongue and use a finger to gently vibrate on either side of the lingual frenulum. (page 113)
- Use verbal reminders to achieve and maintain a "tongue in" positioning.

These techniques will also help reduce drooling. If the child continues to drool, help her learn to discriminate between a "dry mouth" and a "wet mouth." Reinforce her when her mouth is dry. When her mouth is wet, press firmly on the area with a cloth or have the child do it. Remind her to swallow regularly.

Speech Strategies

1. Probe to select speech sound goals. Take into account stimulability as well as which speech sounds most improve intelligibility.

2. After selecting a speech target, think about how the speech sound is made and what the jaw, lips, tongue, soft palate, and air stream need to do to successfully produce the sound. Then observe the child attempting the target sound in various contexts (e.g., isolation, syllables, words, phrases) and see where the system breaks down. Look at the jaw for stability, placement, and shifting. Look at the tongue to see if the appropriate part is making

contact. See if the lips are in position with an appropriate amount of closing, opening, protrusion, and/or retraction. See if the child is producing enough breath support for the speech requirements.

3. Introduce a target speech sound by explaining to the child how the sound is made. Tell her about the specific placement and characteristics in terms she can understand such as tongue and lip placements and movements, vocal fold vibration and opening, and whether the sound is long (sustained/gliding) or short (stop).

4. Increase awareness of the articulator contacts by rubbing the tongue or lips with mouthwash on a cotton swab. Then touch the cotton swab to the point of contact.

5. Put the target speech sound in a phonemic environment that facilitates correct sound placement and production (e.g., when stimulating /w/, precede it with "oo" as in "moo;" the lip position for "oo" is the same one used for "w").

6. The child may need additional time to make articulatory adjustments when using newly learned sounds in syllables and words. If so, segment the syllables or words between the target consonant and the vowel or between syllables during practice (e.g., *b-all, cow-boy*). Gradually shorten the space between the sounds until the word is fully blended.

7. If the child has difficulty with voicing, have her produce the sound while lifting, holding, or carrying a heavy weight such as a therapeutic heavy ball or a chair. The child could also push against the chair back while standing or pull up on the chair seat while seated as she says the sound. She could also hum and then directly produce the sound.

8. If the child has persistent mouth breathing with the jaw open and the tongue in a forward position, refer to a physician for a check of tonsils, adenoids, and allergies. Enlarged tonsils and adenoids and/or the presence of allergies may impede the airway and encourage a more tongue-forward positioning.

9. Regularly monitor hearing and encourage the child's family and physician to treat ear infections and fluid aggressively. Use an FM system or sound amplifier during verbal input to help the child focus on the speaker and process the information.

10. Incorporate repetitive practice of speech targets (i.e., drill) into the therapy sessions.

   a. Children with Down syndrome tend to be reluctant to participate in drill, but they need this repetitive practice of speech skills in order to move to a more automatic level of production.

   b. Structure the therapy sessions to be motivating, rewarding, and fun. Determine the child's interests and incorporate them into therapy activities. Incorporate movement, play, structured action or art activities, games, worksheets, and/or cooking activities into the therapy session for speech drill. It is easier to get repeated practice and review of speech targets by using fun activities along with stickers, practice books with photos, and pictures with written words.

   c. It's important to use spaced, rather than massed practice. Use short periods of practice interspersed with play or structured activities.

11. Use a multisensory cueing approach to teach and cue speech productions.

   a. Multisensory cues utilize several pathways for giving input to the child's sensori-motor and cognitive system. Because the auditory channel is the weakest learning mode for the child with Down syndrome, it's important to utilize the visual-tactile-kinesthetic channels when cueing speech and language.

   b. Multisensory cues include auditory, visual, tactile (touch), and kinesthetic/proprioceptive (movement/feedback). This includes verbal models, amplification, written sounds or words, watching the speaker's face, mirror work, pictures, objects, touch cues (oral-motor facilitation), gross motor movements, pairing sounds with movements, hand signal movements, and verbal and movement feedback.

   c. Use movement activities, movement to rhythm, and/or melodic intonation (i.e., producing speech to rhythm) during production of sounds, syllables, words, or connected speech to facilitate productions as needed.

   d. Use hand signals to represent each consonant sound during speech practice for visual, kinesthetic, and/or tactile cues. You and the child can both use these to facilitate accurate sound production. The hand signals are illustrated and described in Appendix B, *Consonant Hand Signals*, pages 115–117.

   e. Provide all the needed cues to help the child be successful. Then begin to fade them until the child can produce the targets without them.

12. Augment speech with total communication systems.

   a. Use sign, pictures, and written words to augment oral speech.

   b. Make a photo picture book for repeated practice of target words and as a communication aid. This allows the child to create a core vocabulary while still working on sounds or syllable shapes. Write captions or words under the pictures to increase reading skills and incorporate the visual modality. Include pictures of:

   - the child, her family, her house, her pets, her favorite places, her favorite toys, etc.
   - the child with objects or people or doing an action
   - classmates, friends, teachers, and neighbors for a "My Friends" section

   c. For school-aged children, make a "dictionary" language book for the teacher and child to use in the classroom. Think about what the child really needs to be able to communicate (e.g., feelings, wants, preferences, needs, objects, actions, people). Include salient school vocabulary and phrases. Use pictures for the non-reading child.

The child can use this book to clarify what she is trying to communicate, and/or the teacher can use it to gain additional cues.

For children with limited speech, use a communication notebook that goes between school and home. Parents can write about or put in pictures of things that are relevant to the child such as experiences she's had that she may want to relate to teachers and peers. The teacher can write about or put in pictures of things that happened at school.

Select speech words or phrases for the child to practice based on these experiences and print them on the relevant page of the communication book. This provides the child a means for communicating her daily experiences. Key words or phrases may be used for repeated practice as her book is reviewed.

13. No matter the level of intelligibility, respond to the communications as meaningful to teach the power of communication and to increase the desire to communicate verbally.

    a. Give the child communicative ability early by assigning meaning to vocalizations and verbalizations such as isolated speech sounds, syllables, and word approximations (e.g., when the child babbles "Da," you indicate Daddy; if the child says "mmm" or "mo" while eating, you say "more" and give her more).

    b. Rephrase, restate, or provide a correct speech model as needed.

14. Gradually build the child's speech performance load by adding to the length of complexity of the speech production. When building performance load from one- or two-syllable words to multiple-syllable words or from one-word to multiple-word utterances, the following techniques are suggested. Gradually fade these techniques as the child is able to accurately produce the target more naturally.

    a. Use movement on each syllable or word (e.g., clapping).

    b. Use forward, backward, or a variety of chaining.

       • forward chaining: produce the initial syllable of the word several times, then add the second syllable (e.g., "cow, cow, <u>cow</u>boy")
       • backward chaining: produce the final syllable of the word several times, then add the initial syllable (e.g., "boy, boy, cow<u>boy</u>")
       • a variety of chaining in phrases where the ending consonant in the first word becomes the initial sound in the second word (e.g., "look here" becomes "loo-khere")

    c. Write the target word/phrase on cards, worksheets, under pictures, etc. Underline each syllable/word with a different color ink.

    d. Use objects such as blocks or a train engine and cars to represent each syllable or word in a sequence.

    e. Use rhythm, movement, changing stress, pitch, or loudness (e.g., putting emphasis on one word in a phrase by making it louder).

    f. Pause between the syllables or words. Gradually reduce the length of the pause.

    g. Attach a gesture to a targeted utterance or phrase to get some automated speech productions (e.g., shake finger for "bad dog").

    h. Gradually build in prosody, syntax, and pragmatic skills at each level of practice (e.g., to introduce prosody, have the child produce target words with an exclamation or question inflection).

15. Teach some automatic speech (e.g., useful words or phrases like "need help" or "go home").

16. Begin syntax practice when the child begins producing two-word utterances.

17. Use a communication book with the parents to let them know of current goals and objectives, progress, therapy strategies, concerns, or anecdotes about their child. The book can also be used for the parents to communicate progress or concerns with you.

Therapy Sequence from Sounds to Connected Speech

Because of the complex nature of speech disorders in Down syndrome, it is important to use an integrated therapy approach (i.e., selecting techniques from phonology, articulation, dysarthria or oral-motor facilitation, apraxia, and aural rehabilitation therapy).

Information about prerequisites for speech and expressive language and early sound production is found in Chapter 7, pages 61–63. This chapter includes information on establishing joint attention and interaction and facilitating imitation skills.

It's important to understand the general learning styles of children with Down syndrome in order to facilitate speech practice and learning. It may be difficult to get some children to practice, to repeat, to make multiple attempts at a word or sound, and to drill on speech tasks. Remember to take into account that delayed processing, particularly of auditory information, is a characteristic in Down syndrome development. For this reason it's important to give the children additional time to respond and to use multisensory cues for input. Children who perceive speech tasks as difficult can refuse, act out, or use party behavior (e.g., acting cute, performing entertaining actions, etc.), to avoid speech practice. By making the therapy interesting, there will be better cooperation.

Lay the foundation for successful speech production. Use movement, positioning, and oral-motor facilitation to establish sounds as needed. Once the child is at the syllable level and beyond, use a phonological, articulation, or motor-planning approach, depending on the child's needs while continuing to provide movement, positioning, and oral-motor support.

Prerequisites to Speech Practice: Establishing Early Sound Productions

The majority of information on developing prerequisites to production of meaningful speech is found in Chapter 3, pages 25–33 and Chapter 7, pages 61–63. The following are the general prerequisites.

1. Establish rapport.
2. Establish joint attention and interaction.
3. Establish imitation of actions and verbalizations (i.e., pair sounds with actions).

   - Blow bubbles; then interrupt play and have the child imitate "b" for more *bubbles* or "p" to *pop* bubbles.
   - Imitate action-sound combinations like making car sounds while pushing a car; saying "wee" as the child comes down a slide; or presenting an edible treat, rubbing the child's tummy, and saying "mmm."

4. Establish an immediate way to communicate through shaping current vocalizations and verbalizations into meaningful communications. The benefits of this include:

   - validation of the child's attempts to communicate
   - reinforcing her attempts
   - allowing her to operate on her environment
   - teaching the child the power of words
   - accepting the child's present mode of communication and shaping it into recognizable words

Teach the use of key words that are immediately useful and important to the child. Use words with easy motoric productions. Accept approximations. This lets the child know that she is producing words, and it lets the child's family know that the child is using words and making progress.

Therapy Approaches

It's important to combine different types of therapy approaches due to the complexity of the speech disorder in the child with Down syndrome.

1. Phonological Approach

   This therapy approach emphasizes increasing the child's awareness and use of sounds in words. This approach is effective for the unintelligible child who demonstrates a linguistic base to her speech disorder and has patterns of sound errors. It focuses on these patterns instead of on individual sound errors. (See Hodson and Paden, 1991 for more information about a phonological approach.)

a. Select a phonological pattern that the child needs to develop to become more intelligible. Begin with stimulable sounds.

b. Systematically target all sound patterns the child has difficulty with throughout a cycle of intervention (i.e., until all patterns of error are targeted at the word level). During each cycle, cover all patterns of error, concentrating on one at a time. At the end of each cycle, test or probe for mastery of speech sounds and patterns. During the next cycle, again target all error patterns. Follow this with practice of target sounds in phrases and sentences.

c. The most common patterns of error, or phonological processes, are consonant sequence reduction; pre- or post-vocalic singleton consonant omissions (e.g., "cu__" for "cup"); and error patterns on stridents, velars, liquids, nasals, and glides. Other error patterns may be noted (e.g., sound transpositions, stopping).

2. Articulation Approach

This approach is useful when the child needs to remediate specific errors rather than patterns of errors. Components of an articulation approach are:

a. ear training, self-monitoring, and discrimination
b. production of the target sound in isolation
c. production of the sound in syllables
d. production of the sound in words, first in the initial position, then the final position, then in the middle position of words; consonant blends are also targeted
e. production of the sound or blend in phrases or sentences
f. carryover of the sound or blend into conversational speech

3. Dysarthria Approach (Oral-Motor Facilitation)

This is a direct intervention approach that focuses on the sensorimotor system. It is useful for the child with low tone and who has difficulty with precision, strength, steadiness, accuracy, and coordination of the speech system. This approach is used to normalize muscular and postural tone, normalize oral sensitivity, facilitate respiration/ phonation/breath support for speech, and facilitate accurate placements and movements of the articulators. It focuses on the underlying skills necessary for accurate speech production. (See Strode and Chamberlain, 1997 for more information about an oral-motor facilitation approach.)

4. Apraxia Approach (Motor Planning)

This approach emphasizes sound and syllable sequencing and gradually builds the complexity of speech difficulty. It is effective for the child who has difficulty with the motor speech system including motor planning, sound sequencing, and speech production. (See Strode and Chamberlain, 1993 and 1994 for more information about a motor planning/apraxia approach.)

The principal components for this approach are:

a. Gradually build performance load by progressing from production of isolated sounds to syllables, syllable strings, words, multisyllabic words, and finally to connected speech.

b. Work on tasks at different levels simultaneously in the therapy hierarchy (e.g., while working on /m/ in words, also work on other consonant sounds at the syllable level). Use repetitive practice and review at each level in order to habituate new patterns.

c. Use multisensory cues, especially visual-tactile-kinesthetic cues (e.g., hand signals representing each speech sound).

d. Use a vocal warm-up prior to speech practice (e.g., producing all of the long vowels in a sequence).

e. At each level of the progression, place the mastered syllables or words into short phrases. Incorporate prosody techniques. This will increase intelligibility in connected speech.

Have the child produce isolated vowel sounds, vowel sequences, and isolated consonants. Begin vowel and consonant practice with sounds the child can already produce to stabilize productions. Eventually begin to stimulate the production of new vowels and consonants so the child can add new sounds to his speech repertoire. Establish production of consonant sounds that use different places of production such as bilabial, alveolar, and velar.

Put the established vowel and consonant sounds into meaningful context during play or an activity to give the child an immediate way to communicate.

When the child has stabilized several isolated vowel and consonant sounds, teach her how to volitionally, efficiently, and consistently produce syllables using these sounds.

- Begin with consonant-vowel and vowel-consonant sequences. This introduces progressively more complex tasks.
- Combine the syllables into strings by sequencing a consonant-vowel combination into strings of two to three reduplicated syllables (e.g., "meemee," "momo," "moomoomoo").
- Have the child produce consonant-vowel-consonant-vowel syllable sequences with changes in either the consonant or the vowel (e.g., "meemoo" or "meebee").
- Have the child produce consonant-vowel-consonant sequences.
  ▶ Use mastered consonant-vowel or vowel-consonant syllables and add a final or initial consonant to close the syllable (e.g., when the child has mastered the syllable "ba," add an ending sound to make words such as *bab* and *bat*).
  ▶ Begin with consonant-vowel-consonant productions that have the same consonant at the beginning and the end of the word (e.g., *Mom*).
  ▶ Progress to consonant-vowel-consonant words with different consonants in each

position of the word so that the child learns to shift from one articulatory position to another within a word (e.g., *back, bus*).

- Have the child produce multisyllabic words, gradually building the performance load from two-syllable words to words with three to five syllables.

- Then have the child produce consonant blends. Gradually build to multisyllabic words.

- Practice syllables and words in short phrases, expanding to sentences.

5. Aural Rehabilitation Approach

This approach will help the child with a hearing impairment improve her communication abilities. It uses multisensory cues and amplification to enhance the information the child receives. Strategies include the following:

- enhanced use of residual hearing
- speechreading or lipreading
- oral speech training (i.e., teaching the child to produce sounds and words orally using speech)
- kinesthetic methods to develop awareness of speech movements (e.g., hopping while producing the /p/ sound)
- cued speech
- fingerspelling and sign language
- grammar and syntax training
- Total Communication using any or all communication methods available

Selecting Speech Sound Targets

The general sequence of easiest to more difficult types of sounds to produce are bilabials, alveolars, velars, stridents, affricatives, and clusters. Take the following into account when choosing a speech sound or group of sounds for remediation.

- the child's stimulability
- sounds which would most improve her intelligibility
- the presence of low tone or poor oral-motor skills

- apraxia of speech
- hearing loss
- the motor-planning requirements for the sound
- the typical developmental sequence of sound acquisition
- the most frequently occurring sounds that would increase intelligibility most rapidly (e.g., /t, d, n/, with /d/ being the most commonly-occurring sound in English speech)
- the sounds that are most visible (e.g., /m, b, p, w, f, v, t, d, n, sh, ch, j, l, th/)
- speech sounds made at different places of articulation (e.g., bilabials, velars, alveolars); this will facilitate movement patterns as the sounds are combined into syllables and words

---

Typical Developmental Sequence of Sound Acquisition

Generally, children are using sounds in at least one position of words at the following ages (Nicolosi, Harryman, Kresheck, 1989).

3 years: /m, b, p, w, t, d, n, k, g, h, f/

3 1/2 years: /s, z, y/

4 years: /v, j, l, r/

4 1/2 years: /ch/

6 years: /th/

Specific Sequence for Each Therapy Session

Following a systematic plan and sequentially preparing all of the systems for maximum performance leads the child to successful speech production.

1. Prepare the Body

   a. Prepare the body for speech production via a whole body movement or gross motor activity. This helps facilitate/promote alertness, cooperation, muscle and postural tone, respiration/breath support, postural stability and mobility, and prepares the sensory systems for tasks requiring attention.

   Use specific movements to help stimulate specific types of sounds. Suggested activities for stop or plosive sounds are short bursts of movement (e.g., jumping, punching, skipping, bouncing, kicking, hopping, or pounding).

   Suggested activities for continuant and liquid sounds are long, sustained movements (e.g., sliding, swinging, rolling, skating, squeezing, pulling). Other types of sustained movements include resistance activities (e.g., pulling on a rope, hanging on a rope, pushing a heavy box, carrying a heavy object). Sustained blowing or resistive sucking through a straw are also suggested.

   Incorporate respiration/phonation/breath control activities within gross motor activities or other appropriate activities (e.g., aerobic exercise like running).

   b. Position the child appropriately for oral-motor facilitation and speech activities.

2. Prepare the Oral Mechanism Outside the Mouth

   Prepare the oral mechanism for speech tasks starting outside the mouth, on the face. Techniques include face pats, massage, vibration, rubbing, stroking, stretching, sustained blowing, and resistive sucking. (See Appendix A, pages 106–114.)

3. Normalize Oral Sensitivity

   Normalize sensitivity in the oral area to decrease tactile defensiveness and increase sensory awareness. (See pages 84–85.)

4. Reduce Habitual Tongue Protrusion Pattern

   Use positioning, touch input, and verbal reminders to reduce the tongue protrusion pattern. (See pages 87–88.)

5. Prepare the Oral Mechanism Inside the Mouth

    Use direct oral facilitation techniques to the articulators to facilitate production of individual speech sounds as needed. These direct touch techniques facilitate sensory awareness in the oral area; help normalize tone and sensitivity, muscle strength and precision; coordination of movements; and volitional control of articulator positioning/oral movement. They are listed on pages 96–104 for each group of speech sounds.

    Speech facilitation activities should always be followed by a functional task (e.g., eating, speech work). Food experiences can be a less intrusive way of beginning work inside the mouth.

6. Warm Up the Speech System

    Warm up the speech mechanism through imitations of speech and environmental sounds, including sustained productions of each long vowel in a sequence.

7. Speech Performance and Practice

    Use a phonological, articulation, or motor-planning based approach to speech remediation, or elements from each as appropriate. Use the following routine during each session:

    a. vocal warm-up, including production of speech or environmental sounds

    b. review of previous speech targets

    c. introduction of new speech targets (use multisensory cues and oral-motor facilitation techniques as needed)

    d. systematic rehearsal and drill (i.e., Model the sound, syllable, or word. Practice it with the child, then have her produce it. Repeat.)

    e. incorporate speech targets into real activities to give them meaning; this allows the child to generalize their use

For more practice, put the speech targets into a speech practice book for review and home practice (e.g., pictures, printed words).

Use the target productions to communicate a variety of functions such as requesting, commenting, greeting (social words), questioning, and refusing/protesting. Structure the environment so the child has to use these words. Use natural communication prompts to facilitate pragmatics (e.g., "What do you want?").

8. Use Multisensory Cues

    Use multisensory cues along with direct touch techniques, particularly the hand signals for each consonant sound. This will help in the transition from production of isolated sounds to sound sequencing.

    Illustrations and descriptions of the hand signals are found in Appendix B, pages 115–117. (For more information about oral-motor facilitation of speech, see Strode and Chamberlain, 1997.)

Speech Sound Groups and Specific Intervention for Each

Direct oral-motor facilitation techniques can be applied to the articulators to facilitate accurate production of speech sounds. The specific sounds are presented in groups based on the production features of the sounds.

Not all direct techniques listed under a sound group must be used. Select the ones that facilitate the child's articulator placement for the target speech sound. Generally repeat each technique three times. Be sure to position the child correctly and to apply techniques symmetrically to both sides of the face, jaw, lips, and tongue.

When the child can produce the target speech sound voluntarily with consistency, direct techniques may be faded.

Not all of the direct oral-motor facilitation techniques are described under each sound group. The starred (*)

techniques are described and illustrated in Appendix A, pages 106–114.

To make oral-motor facilitation easier, make an oral-motor therapy equipment box that contains all the necessary supplies. Suggested materials:

- latex gloves
- blowing toys (e.g., horns, whistles, party blowers)
- cotton swabs
- edible treats (e.g., raisins, dried fruit, peanut butter)
- dental floss and dental floss holders
- straws
- aquarium tubing (clear plastic tubing of different diameters available at pet stores)
- Infa-dents®
- toothbrushes
- Toothettes®
- mouthwash
- coffee stirrers
- blunt flat toothpicks
- tongue depressors
- washcloth
- rubbing alcohol
- antibacterial soap

Clean oral-motor equipment well. Use an antibacterial soap and rinse well or clean with rubbing alcohol. Some items may be cleaned in the dishwasher on the top shelf. Wear gloves and wash well when working on the child's face or in the mouth. Check the child for latex allergies before using gloves.

Labial Sounds /p, b, m, w/

Children with Down syndrome often have difficulty with labial sounds. Factors that contribute to the difficulty include the following:

- hypotonia throughout the body which can result in poor postural alignment of the body
- poor jaw stability and grading with slack open jaw, poor jaw alignment, and mouth breathing
- low tone in the lips and face
- reduced lip strength
- poor awareness of articulator contact
- reduced respiration/phonation and air pressure buildup due to leaky vocal folds and/or poor lip seal resulting in weak production of bilabials

Each of the following direct techniques for facilitating sound placement are appropriate to facilitate /p, b/ and /m/. Techniques 4 through 6 are appropriate to facilitate /w/.

1. To increase sensory awareness of lip contact, rub the contact surfaces of the upper and lower lip with texture (e.g., washcloth, toothbrush) or a cotton swab dipped in mouthwash.

2. Put a washcloth, straw, or a tongue depressor flat between the child's lips. Have her resist as you gently attempt to pull it out. Make sure the object is between the lips only, not the child's teeth.

3. Have the child briefly suck on ice cubes or a Popsicle®.

4. Do bunny nose*, V-pressure*, mustache press*, lip stroke*, pucker resistance*, and/or smile resistance* exercises. (pages 108 and 109)

5. Apply sustained blowing activities*. (Note: Use larger straws or plastic aquarium tubing to facilitate lip rounding for /w/.) (page 114)

6. Apply resistive sucking activities*. (page 114)

Labiodental Sounds /f, v/

Children with Down syndrome often have difficulty with labiodental sounds. Factors that contribute to the difficulty include the following:

- hypotonia throughout the body which can result in poor postural alignment of the body
- poor jaw stability and grading with slack open jaw, poor jaw alignment, and mouth breathing
- low tone in the lips and face
- protrusion pattern of the tongue
- reduced lip strength
- poor awareness of articulator contacts
- reduced respiration/phonation and buildup of air pressure at the lips or larynx

Each of the following direct techniques for facilitating sound placement are appropriate to facilitate /f/ and /v/.

1. To increase sensory awareness, use the fingers to tap along the lower lip four or five times gently, but firmly. Do the same on the bottom edge of the upper central incisors. This may be done with a stroke using a cotton swab dipped into mouthwash or a washcloth.

2. Apply lip stroke* to the bottom lip only. (page 109)

3. Place the index finger along the entire lower lip. Apply deep pressure into the lip and hold for four to five seconds. Then use your fingers to apply sustained pressure to the upper teeth.

4. Manually tuck the child's lower lip into her mouth while providing jaw support. With the child's teeth open slightly, gently press upward with your finger as you push the child's lip into her mouth between her teeth.

5. Have the child briefly suck an ice cube or Popsicle®. Rub the ice on the child's lower lip and on the edge of the child's upper teeth.

6. Have the child use her front teeth to bite through carrot or celery sticks or crackers to encourage appropriate jaw function.

7. Put peanut butter or another sticky food on the child's lower lip and have her scrape it off using her upper teeth.

Lingua-Alveolar Sounds /t, d, n/

Children with Down syndrome often have difficulty with lingua-alveolar sounds. Factors that contribute to the difficulty include the following:

- hypotonia throughout the body which can result in poor postural alignment of the body
- lack of good jaw-tongue separation for independent movement of the tongue
- poor jaw stability and grading with slack open jaw, poor jaw alignment, and mouth breathing
- low tone in the face, lips, and tongue
- positioning of the tongue forward and flat with reduced tone; tendency to use a front-back movement of the tongue rather than a more mature movement pattern with grooving, elevation, and tension
  - a. reduced precise tongue movement and contact
  - b. reduced elevation of tongue front and sides
  - c. reduced tongue tension and strength
- poor awareness of articulator contacts
- reduced respiration/phonation and air pressure buildup due to leaky vocal folds and/or poor tongue seal resulting in weak production of /t/ and /d/ which are produced more as continuants than plosives

Each of the following direct techniques for facilitating sound placement are appropriate to facilitate /t, d/ and /n/.

1. To increase sensory awareness, rub the sides and tip of the tongue and the alveolar ridge with texture (e.g., washcloth, toothbrush, cotton swab, Infadent®, or Toothette®) as you name the points of contact.

2. Use your finger to apply deep pressure to the tongue front and tip in a series of quick taps.

3. Do tongue tip press: in*, tongue tip press: down*, tongue tip press: lateral*, and/or tongue stroke* exercises. (pages 110, 111, and 113)

4. With your gloved finger, press down on the front top of the child's tongue at the center. Slowly lift your finger and ask the child to follow your finger with her tongue.

5. Hold a sucker, pretzel, carrot stick, celery stick, tongue blade, or Popsicle® upright in front of the child's mouth. Have her use her tongue to lick from the bottom to the top of the object without moving her head.

6. Put a thin cocktail straw or coffee stirrer horizontally behind the child's front teeth (i.e., side-to-side, not front-to-back). Have her hold it there for a count of 10 using only the front of her tongue. Don't let her close down her jaw to hold the straw.

7. Place a sticky food on the child's alveolar ridge. Have her lick it off with the front and tip of her tongue using a front-to-back motion rather than a sucking motion.

Velar Sounds /k, g/

Children with Down syndrome often have difficulty with velar sounds. Factors that contribute to the difficulty include the following:

- hypotonia throughout the body which can result in poor postural alignment of the body
- lack of good jaw-tongue separation for independent movement of the tongue
- poor jaw stability and grading with slack open jaw, poor jaw alignment, and mouth breathing
- low tone in the face, lips, and tongue
- positioning of the tongue forward and flat with reduced tone; tendency to use a front-back movement of the tongue rather than a more mature movement pattern with grooving, elevation, and tension
     a. reduced tension and tone in the tongue
     b. reduced retraction of the tongue
- poor awareness of articulator contacts
- reduced respiration/phonation and air pressure buildup due to leaky vocal folds and/or poor tongue seal

Each of the following direct techniques for facilitating sound placement are appropriate to facilitate /k/ and /g/.

I. To increase sensory awareness, rub the sides of the back half of the child's tongue, moving from front to back with a finger, Toothette®, Infa-dent®, or a cotton swab dipped in mouthwash. Then rub the insides of the back teeth along the gum edge.

2. Do central groove tap*, tongue back press: top*, tongue back press: sides*, and/or tongue base press* exercises. (pages 110 – 112)

3. Have the child drink a tart liquid such as lemonade or cranberry juice through a thin straw.

Lingua-Alveolar Strident Sounds /s, z/

Children with Down syndrome often have difficulty with strident sounds. Factors that contribute to the difficulty include the following:

- hypotonia throughout the body which can result in poor postural alignment of the body
- lack of good jaw-tongue separation for independent movement of the tongue
- poor jaw stability and grading with slack open jaw, poor jaw alignment, and mouth breathing
- low tone in the face, lips, and tongue
- positioning of the tongue forward and flat with reduced tone; tendency to use a front-back movement of the tongue rather than a more mature movement pattern with grooving, elevation, and tension
     a. reduced tongue groove
     b. reduced elevation of tongue front and sides
     c. reduced tongue tension and strength
- poor awareness of articulator contacts
- reduced respiration/phonation and air pressure buildup

There are several important factors that can affect placement and production of /s/ and /z/. Direct techniques for sound placement are listed in a general therapy progression to target these factors. Techniques to facilitate jaw stability, a central groove in the tongue, and elevation of the tongue tip and sides are listed below. Select techniques as needed for a frontal lisp, a lateral lisp, or for increased respiration/breath support for these sounds. Some techniques may target more than one problem area.

I. Facilitate jaw stability and graded jaw movements. Without this control, the tongue has difficulty moving independently to find and maintain a correct position for sound production. Jaw positioning, stability, and control can be affected by overall body positioning, body and facial muscle tone, and by a habitual jaw-open position with mouth breathing.

     a. Use jaw resistance activities*. (page 107)
     b. Do the push into the point of the chin* exercise. (page 108)
     c. Apply biting and chewing activities.

d. Do sustained blowing* and resistive sucking* activities. (page 114)

e. Use a bite block* to stabilize the jaw and maintain a jaw opening without shifting or excessive opening during speech attempts. (page 108)

f. Use jaw cupping* or position the child's chin on her fist during speech productions as needed. (page 108)

2. Facilitate a central groove in the midline of the tongue to get tongue placement and proper airflow. The central groove is needed for passage of the air stream. When the air stream is absent or reduced, the child omits the /s/ or /z/ or substitutes a stop, a lateral production, or a frontal production.

a. Use central groove stroke* and/or central groove tap* exercises. (page 110)

b. Put a thin straw, a flat blunt toothpick, or a coffee stirrer on the front quarter of the central groove of the child's tongue. Have the child produce a sustained /s/ with the object on the central groove. Slowly pull the object out as the child continues to blow air and produce the sound.

3. Facilitate elevation of the tongue tip and sides. An elevated tongue tip with a central groove and front opening for airflow is needed, although some children may be more successful with the tongue tip depressed. Without elevation of the sides of the tongue, the sound may be produced as a stop or with lateralized airflow.

a. To increase sensory awareness, use your gloved finger or texture (e.g., pretzel, washcloth, Infa-dent®, Toothette®) to rub the alveolus and the tongue where contact is made between the two. Name the parts.

b. Stroke each side of the tip of the tongue. Begin at the center of the tip and stroke one quarter of the way back on each side of the tongue. Then stroke each top side of the tongue along the edges from the tip to the back.

c. Do tongue tip press: in* and/or tongue tip press: down* exercises. (page 110)

d. Do tongue side press: in*. Repeat and have the child push back with her tongue (resistance). (page 112)

e. Do tongue side press: down*. Repeat as the child attempts to push up (resistance). (page 112)

f. Place a sticky food such as peanut butter, jelly, icing from a tube, or marshmallow cream on the center of the child's alveolus and have her lick it off, using the front and tip of her tongue to lick from front to back.

4. Counteract excessive tongue protrusion (frontal lisp). The tongue needs to be retracted behind the central incisors.

a. Apply jaw techniques* as needed. (pages 107 and 108)

b. Apply central groove techniques*. (page 110)

c. Use tongue stroke* along with tongue tip and side elevation techniques* from above. Stroke the tongue on the midline from the center to the tip. (page 113)

d. Grasp the child's tongue with a washcloth, pull it forward, briefly hold it, then release it.

e. Elevate the child's tongue and briefly vibrate on either side of the lingual frenum.

f. Do resistive sucking through a straw*. Put the straw on the front central groove (midline of the tongue) when drinking. The child's tongue should be in her mouth, not protruded. Use a tart drink such as lemonade or cranberry juice to facilitate tongue retraction. (page 114)

5. Counteract lateral emission of airflow (lateralized production). The sides of the tongue must be elevated and there must be a central groove for airflow for a non-lateralized strident production.

a. Apply jaw techniques* as needed. (pages 107 and 108)

b. Apply central groove techniques*. In a lateral production, the air tends to flow over the sides of the tongue rather than down the central groove. (page 110)

c. Apply tongue tip and side elevation techniques*. Emphasize elevation of the sides of the tongue. (pages 110–113)

d. Use a bite block* during speech to stabilize the jaw and maintain mouth opening without shifting or excessive opening of the jaw. (page 108)

6. Facilitate respiration/breath support for speech. Without appropriate air support for speech, the

strident may become an omission or stop, and there may be cluster or syllabication reduction.

a. See gross motor movement techniques under Prepare the Body, page 94.
b. Position the child with the head, neck, and hips in alignment.
c. Do blowing activities* that require sustained breath. (page II4)
d. The child may lie on her stomach, propped on her elbows during speech production.
e. Have the child produce sustained vowels, a continuous vowel sequence, or sustained vowels gliding into a strident production (e.g., "eeesss").
f. Push into the child's diaphragm as she produces the strident sound.
g. Do exercises that facilitate breath control such as jumping, bouncing, running, sit-ups, or yoga.
h. Have the child lie facedown over a large therapy ball. Hold the child at the hips. Push into the ball as you bounce her.

7. Counteract substitution of a stop sound for the continuant.

a. Apply jaw techniques* as needed. (pages I07 and I08)
b. Apply central groove techniques*. (page II0)
c. Try an alternate placement (i.e., the tongue tip down).
d. Use techniques to facilitate elevation and spreading of the lateral margins of the tongue. Do tongue side press: in*, tongue side press: down*, and/or tongue spread* exercises. (pages II2 and II3)
e. Work on respiration and breath support for speech.

Palatal Sounds /sh, ch, j/

Children with Down syndrome often have difficulty with palatal sounds. Factors that contribute to the difficulty include the following:

- hypotonia throughout the body which can result in poor postural alignment of the body
- lack of good jaw-tongue separation for independent movement of the tongue
- poor jaw stability and grading with slack open jaw, poor jaw alignment, and mouth breathing

- low tone in the face, lips, and tongue
- positioning of the tongue forward and flat with reduced tone; tendency to use a front-back movement of the tongue rather than a more mature movement pattern with grooving, elevation, and tension
    a. reduced tongue groove
    b. reduced elevation of tongue front and sides
    c. reduced tongue tension and strength
- poor awareness of articulator contacts
- reduced respiration/phonation and air pressure buildup
- reduced plosive nature of /ch/ and /j/

There are several important factors that can affect placement and production of /sh, ch/ and /j/. Direct techniques for sound placement are listed in a general therapy progression to target these factors. Techniques to facilitate jaw stability, a central groove in the tongue, and elevation of the tongue tip and sides are listed below and on the next page. Select additional techniques as needed to target a frontal or lateral production or respiration/ breath support for these sounds. Some techniques may target more than one problem area.

I. Facilitate jaw stability and graded jaw movements*. Without this control, the tongue has difficulty moving independently to find and maintain a correct position for sound production. Jaw positioning, stability, and control can be affected by overall body positioning, body and facial muscle tone, and by a habitual jaw-open position with mouth breathing.

a. Apply jaw resistance activities*. (page I07)
b. Do the push into the point of the chin* exercise. (page I08)
c. Apply biting and chewing activities.
d. Do sustained blowing* and resistive sucking* activities. (page II4)
e. Use a bite block* to stabilize the jaw and maintain a jaw opening without shifting or excessive opening during speech attempts. (page I08)
f. Use jaw cupping* or position the child's chin on her fist during speech productions as needed. (page I08)

2. Facilitate a central groove in the midline of the tongue to get tongue placement and proper airflow.

This is needed for the passage of the airstream. When it is absent or reduced, the child produces the strident frontally, laterally, omits it, or substitutes a stop for it.

    a. Do central groove stroke* exercise. (page 110)
    b. Do central groove tap* exercise. (page 110)

3. Facilitate elevation of the tongue tip and sides and spreading of the tongue. An elevated tongue tip with a central groove and front opening for airflow is needed. Without spreading and elevation of the sides of the tongue, the production may be a stop, a frontal production, or a lateral production.

    a. To increase sensory awareness, stroke the top sides of the tongue from the tip to the back, first stroking one side, then the other.
    b. Do tongue tip press: in*, tongue tip press: down*, and/or tongue tip press: lateral* exercises. (pages 110 and 111)
    c. Do tongue side press: in*. Repeat and have the child push back with her tongue (resistance). (page 112)
    d. Do tongue side press: down.* Push down as the child attempts to push up (resistance). Don't let her use her head to help. (page 112)
    e. Do tongue spread* exercise. (page 113)
    f. Encourage elevation of the back sides of the tongue using techniques a, b, and c.

4. Counteract excessive tongue protrusion (interdental placement).

    a. Apply jaw resistance techniques*. (page 107)
    b. Apply central groove techniques*. (page 110)
    c. Do tongue stroke* exercise. (page 113)
    d. Tap the tongue tip and front using short quick taps.
    e. Apply tongue tip and side elevation techniques.* (pages 110 – 113)
    f. Grasp the child's tongue with a washcloth, pull it forward, and briefly hold it.
    g. Elevate the child's tongue and briefly vibrate on either side of the lingual frenum.
    h. Use a bite block* during speech to stabilize the jaw and maintain jaw opening without shifting or excessive opening. (page 108)

5. Counteract lateral emission of airflow (lateralized production). The sides of the tongue must be elevated and there must be a central groove for airflow for a non-lateralized strident production. If the child lateralizes a palatal sound, work on increased lip rounding, central groove of the tongue, elevation of the lateral margins of the tongue, and jaw position and stability.

    a. Apply jaw resistance techniques*. (page 107)
    b. Apply central groove techniques*. In a lateral production, the air tends to flow over the sides of the tongue rather than down the central groove. (page 110)
    c. Apply tongue tip and side elevation techniques. Emphasize elevation of the sides of the tongue. (pages 110 – 113)
    d. Use a bite block* during speech to stabilize the jaw and maintain jaw opening without shifting or excessive opening. Apply other jaw stability and control techniques as needed. (page 108)

6. Increase lip tension to facilitate rounding.

    a. Do sustained blowing activities* or resistive sucking*. (page 114)
    b. Do manual vibration to the facial muscles, particularly around the lips*. (page 107)
    c. Do lip stroke*, pucker resistance*, and/or smile resistance* exercises. (page 109)

7. Facilitate respiration/air support for /sh, ch/ and /j/. Without appropriate air support for speech, a stop sound may be substituted for the strident or the strident may be omitted.

    a. See gross motor movement techniques under Prepare the Body, page 94.
    b. Do blowing activities* that require sustained breath. (page 114)
    c. Have the child lie on her stomach, propped on her elbows during speech production.
    d. Produce sustained vowels, a continuous vowel sequence, or sustained vowels gliding into a strident production (e.g., "iiiish").
    e. Push into the child's diaphragm as she produces the strident sound.
    f. Do exercises that facilitate breath control such as jumping, bouncing, running, or sit-ups.

g. Have the child lie facedown over a large therapy ball. Hold the child at the hips. Push into the ball as you bounce her.

h. Make sure the child's head, neck, and hips are in alignment.

8. If the child uses a stop for a continuant, work on placement of the sides of the tongue, airflow, and the central groove and opening at the front of the tongue.

Lingua-Alveolar Glide Sound /l/

Children with Down syndrome often have difficulty with lingua-alveolar glide sound. Factors that contribute to the difficulty include the following:

- hypotonia throughout the body which can result in poor postural alignment of the body
- lack of good jaw-tongue separation for independent movement of the tongue
- poor jaw stability and grading with slack open jaw, poor jaw alignment, and mouth breathing
- low tone in the face, lips, and tongue
- positioning of the tongue forward and flat with reduced tone; tendency to use a front-back movement of the tongue rather than a more mature movement pattern with grooving, elevation, and tension
    a. reduced precise tongue movement and contact
    b. reduced elevation of tongue front
    c. reduced tongue tension and strength
- poor awareness of articulator contacts
- reduced respiration/phonation and air pressure buildup due to leaky vocal folds and/or poor tongue seal

Each of the following direct techniques for facilitating sound placement are appropriate to facilitate /l/.

1. To increase sensory awareness, rub the sides and tip of the child's tongue as well as the alveolus with texture (e.g., washcloth, toothbrush, cotton swab, Toothette®, or Infa-dent®) as you name the points of contact.

2. Facilitate jaw stability and graded jaw movements*. Without this control, the tongue has difficulty moving independently to find and maintain a correct position for sound production. Jaw positioning, stability, and control can be affected by overall body positioning, body and facial muscle tone, and by a habitual jaw-open position with mouth breathing.

a. Apply jaw resistance activities*. (page 107)
b. Do the push into the point of the chin* exercise. (page 108)
c. Apply biting and chewing activities.
d. Do sustained blowing* and resistive sucking* activities. (page 114)
e. Use a bite block* to stabilize the jaw and maintain a jaw opening without shifting or excessive opening during speech attempts. (page 108)
f. Use jaw cupping* or position the child's chin on her fist during speech productions as needed. (page 108)

3. Use your finger to apply deep pressure to the tongue front and tip in a series of quick taps.

4. Do tongue tip press: down*, tongue tip press: lateral*, tongue stroke*, and/or tongue tip elevation* exercises. (pages 110, 111, and 113)

5. Press down on the top of the front of the child's tongue at the center with your finger. Slowly lift your finger and ask the child to follow it with her tongue.

6. Hold a sucker, pretzel, carrot stick, celery stick, tongue blade, or Popsicle® upright in front of the child's mouth. Have the child use her tongue to lick from the bottom to the top of the object without moving her head. Repeat, providing proprioceptive input by pulling down on the object as the child licks up.

7. Put a thin cocktail straw or coffee stirrer horizontally (i.e., side-to-side, not front-to-back) behind the child's front teeth. Have her hold it there for a count of 10 using only the front of her tongue. Don't let the child close down her jaw to hold the straw. You can also place the straw on the central groove of the child's tongue and have her hold it against the alveolus.

8. Place a small amount of a sticky food such as peanut butter, jelly, or marshmallow cream on the center of the child's alveolus and palate. Have the child use the front of her tongue to lick from the alveolus back to the palate.

9. If the child is using lip rounding (which encourages substitution of /w/), have her smile slightly. You can also do techniques that encourage lip retraction such as stroking the lips from the center to the corners. Begin with words or syllables that contain the vowel "eee" (e.g., *leak, leap, believe*) which facilitate lip retraction.

Palatal Glide Sounds /r, er/

Children with Down syndrome often have difficulty with /r/ and /er/ sounds. Factors that contribute to the difficulty include the following:

*   hypotonia throughout the body which can result in poor postural alignment of the body
*   lack of good jaw-tongue separation for independent movement of the tongue
*   poor jaw stability and grading with slack open jaw, poor jaw alignment, and mouth breathing
*   low tone in the face, lips, and tongue
*   positioning of the tongue forward and flat with reduced tone; tendency to use a front-back movement of the tongue rather than a more mature movement pattern with grooving, elevation, and tension
    a. reduced precise tongue movement and contact
    b. reduced elevation of the tongue front, sides, and back
    c. reduced tongue tension and strength
*   poor awareness of articulator contacts
*   reduced respiration/phonation and air pressure buildup

These techniques are listed in a general progression to address the key variables for achieving correct /r/ and /er/ placement and production. The techniques under each heading may target more than one element. Not all techniques need to be implemented. You will need to determine which factors are affecting /r/ and /er/ placement difficulty and which areas to address.

1. Facilitate jaw stability and graded jaw movements so that jaw positioning is controlled and the tongue moves independently from the jaw. It's important to check jaw positioning and stability carefully. Many children who distort /er/ have difficulty maintaining a neutral jaw position. They may jut the jaw forward, laterally, or use a lax open jaw which pulls the tongue out of position. Poor postural alignment can affect jaw functioning.

    a. Apply jaw resistance activities*. (page 107)
    b. Do the push into the point of the chin* exercise. (page 110)
    c. Apply biting and chewing activities.
    d. Do sustained blowing* and resistive sucking* activities. (page 114)
    e. Use a bite block* to stabilize the jaw and maintain a jaw opening without shifting or excessive opening during speech attempts. (page 108)
    f. Use jaw cupping* or position the child's chin on her fist during speech productions as needed. (page 108)

2. Facilitate an appropriate amount of tension throughout the tongue.

    a. Do tongue side press: in*. Repeat and have the child push against your finger with her tongue (resistance). (page 112)
    b. Do tongue side press: down*. Repeat with the child using her tongue to push up against your finger (resistance). (page 112)
    c. Push down on the center of the front of the child's tongue with your gloved finger as the child attempts to push your finger up (resistance).
    d. If the child's tongue is overly tense so that she distorts /er/, work on tongue position (spreading and elevation of the back especially), and a reduction of tension in the tongue. It may help to close the jaw down some and produce the /er/ with a rising pitch.
    e. If the child does not have enough tension in the tongue, repeat gross motor and facial movements and inputs, page 94. Then apply the direct techniques from above and those that encourage tongue elevation and spreading.

3. Facilitate tongue retraction. The child's tongue should be pulled back with the back lateral margins elevated.

    a. Using a gloved finger, a cotton swab dipped in mouthwash, a washcloth, an Infa-dent®, or a Toothette®, stroke the sides of the child's tongue and the upper molars and gums. Then have the child raise her tongue so the sides are in contact with the sides of the molars. Have her slowly slide her tongue back, maintaining contact between the sides of the tongue and the molars.
    b. Have the child gently bite the sides of her tongue between her molars as she slides her tongue back.
    c. Put a tongue depressor into the tip of the child's tongue. Push the tongue straight back for the /er/. You can also put the depressor under the front of the child's tongue and push back and slightly up.
    d. Touch the back of the child's head at the base of her skull as she retracts her tongue. You can also gently pull the child's hair back at the base of her skull. These techniques give tactile information about tongue retraction.

4. Facilitate elevation of the back and sides of the tongue, and spreading of the tongue.

    a. To increase sensory awareness, use a gloved finger, a cotton swab dipped in mouthwash, a washcloth, an Infa-dent®, or a Toothette® to stroke the sides of the tongue and the upper molars and gums where contact is made.
    b. Do tongue side press: in*. Repeat and have the child push against your finger with her tongue (resistance). (page 112)
    c. Do tongue side press: down*. Repeat and have the child push up against your finger with her tongue (resistance). (page 112)
    d. Do tongue spread* and/or tongue base press* exercises. (pages 110 and 111)

5. Facilitate a central groove in the midline of the tongue to get tongue placement with the back sides elevated so that the tongue is spoon-shaped.

    a. Do central groove stroke* exercise. (page 110)
    b. Do central groove tap* exercise. (page 110)

6. Facilitate elevation of the tongue tip and front.

    a. Apply deep pressure to the front and tip of the child's tongue in a series of quick taps with the finger.
    b. Do tongue tip press: in*. Repeat with the child pushing against your finger with her tongue tip (resistance). Don't let her push with her head. (page 110)
    c. Do tongue tip press: down*. Push down on the child's tongue as she pushes up (resistance). (page 110)
    d. Do tongue tip press: lateral* applied to the tongue front. Repeat as the child pushes against your finger (resistance). (page 111)
    e. Press down on the front of the center of the child's tongue with your finger. Slowly lift your finger and ask the child to follow it with her tongue.
    f. Put a tongue depressor under or into the tip of the child's tongue. Push the tongue back and slightly up for the /er/. For the retroflex position, push the tongue tip all the way up and back.

7. If the child is substituting /w/ for /r/, encourage lip spreading rather than rounding.

    a. Apply manual vibration* using slow vibration to the face. Slow vibration will reduce facial tension. (page 107)
    b. Stroke the child's lips from the corners to the center, then shake the center gently to reduce lip tension.
    c. Use a lip-spread vowel such as "ee" to precede the /r/ (e.g., *ear, deer, here*).
    d. Use a smile and elongate the /r/ sound.
    e. Use a mirror to monitor lip position.

Consonant Blends
The general sequence of teaching /s, l/ and /r/ blends is as follows:

1. two-element blends in words
2. three-element blends in words
3. blends in phrases and sentences

Apply appropriate techniques from above to facilitate the consonant sounds in the blends.

Prosody

Prosody is the melody of speech; the rhythm, intonation, rate, pitch, loudness, syllable stress, and timing. Children with Down syndrome often lose intelligibility in connected speech due to problems with prosody. Any or all of the following prosody aspects can be impacted in the child with Down syndrome.

- intonation contours (i.e., rising and falling pitches used to denote sentences as declarative, exclamatory, or questions)
- pitch range
- speaking rate
- appropriate separation of syllables and words
- appropriate syllabic and word stress
- intensity levels

Addressing prosody will increase overall speech intelligibility as the child begins producing sentences and connected speech. It's important to introduce prosody and the effects of prosody use early. The child can use pitch variations and suprasegmentals to indicate differences in meaning (e.g., saying a phrase as a sentence vs. a question).

Begin by varying the inflection, varying loudness or pitch, lengthening vowels, and/or adding rhythm. Incorporate songs or fingerplays for the younger child using inflection. Prosody practice frequently should be included in activities as the child develops speech.

Intervention

1. Facilitate appropriate intonation contours and pitch.

   a. Produce utterances as if mad, sad, happy, excited, or afraid. Use a question/declarative contour production.
   b. Help the child make a request or ask a question using intonational and pitch changes, even when at the one-word utterance level.
   c. Use rhythm during speech productions. Melodic intonation techniques are useful (e.g., speaking to rhythm).
   d. Role-play or use scripts using different intonation contours such as questions, emphasis, declarative, imperative, etc. (e.g., role-play a customer in a store and say things like "I need a shirt. Do you have a blue one? I like that one!").

   e. Exaggerate intonational contours to facilitate sound, syllable, word, and phrase segmentations.
   f. Teach and practice key phrases the child will use often. Practice them with appropriate intonation contours.

2. Facilitate the use of a more appropriate rate. Help the child slow down the rate using one or more of the following.

   a. Use a pacing board to help add separations between syllables and words.
   b. Use rhythm, melodic intonation, or talking to a beat.
   c. Use a signal such as the sign for "slow" to cue the child to slow her rate.
   d. Use objects to illustrate rate variations, such as slow and fast moving toy cars.
   e. Model the use of appropriate rate by using a slower rate when talking to the child.

3. Increase the space between words and syllables to help slow rate and increase intelligibility.

4. Use appropriate syllable stress and word stress in phrases and sentences.

   a. Give the older child a statement such as "John is driving the dump truck." Teach the child to emphasize different words in the sentence according to the question asked. Practice using appropriate stress in scripts, role-playing, or in real-life situations.

      - "Is PETE driving the dump truck?" "No, JOHN is driving the dump truck."
      - "Is John PUSHING the dump truck?" "No, John is DRIVING the dump truck."
      - "Is John driving a CAR?" "No, John is driving a DUMP TRUCK."

5. Develop appropriate loudness levels. Increase loudness to emphasize new targets or to stress a word or syllable.

6. Breath support and prosody may be linked. Working on breath support activities along with speech may facilitate prosody.

Appendix A: Illustrated Oral-Motor Techniques

Not all techniques are illustrated. A technique may fall under more than one heading because it may facilitate more than one position or movement.

Positioning

It's important to give the speech mechanism a stable base.

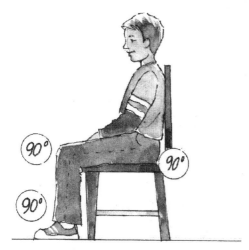

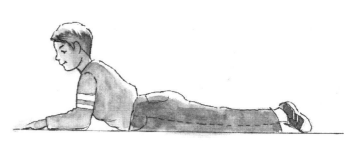

1. **90° - 90° - 90°**
    hips, knees, and ankles at 90°;
    feet flat on floor

2. **prone on elbows**
    elbows directly under shoulders,
    head forward and up
    (not sunk between shoulders)

Face Wake-Ups

This is used to prepare the muscles of the face and mouth for speech production.

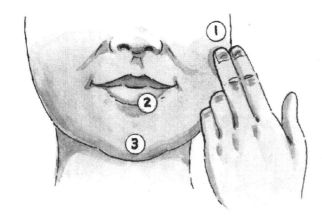

1. **face pats**
    Use two fingers to pat cheeks, lips, and chin.

a.   b.

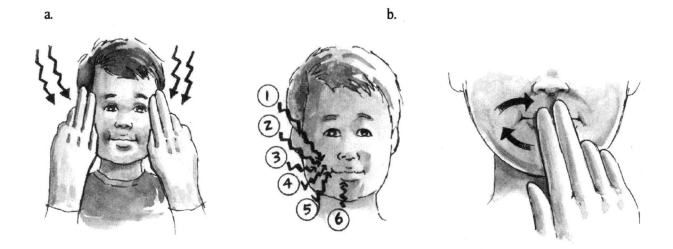

2. **manual vibration**
   Using your index and middle fingers, (a) vibrate along facial muscles from origin to point of insertion at mouth and (b) around lips.

Jaw Stability Techniques

Jaw stability and grading are important for all speech sounds, particularly for connected speech.

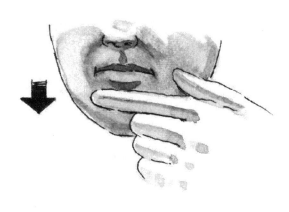

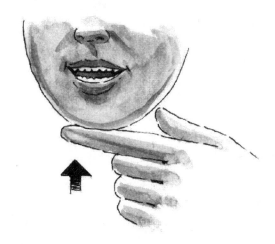

1. **resistance to jaw opening**
   Push down on the child's chin as he attempts to keep his mouth closed.

2. **resistance to jaw closing**
   Push upward on the child's chin while he attempts to keep his mouth open.

107

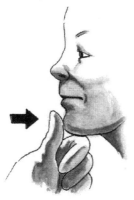

3. push into the point of the chin
Push inward on the point of the child's chin.

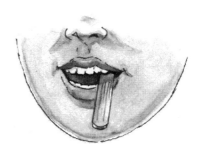

4. bite block
Place an object between the child's molars.

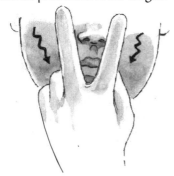

5. jaw cupping
Have the child cup his chin between the palms of both hands with his fingers along his jaw and his thumbs along or behind the angle of the mandible.

Lip Closure Techniques

These techniques are important for /p, b/ and /m/ sounds. Lip closure can be affected by head and back positioning, low tone, stability, and habitual protrusion of the tongue.

I. bunny nose
Place your index and middle fingers on either side of the child's nose. Vibrate down to the child's top lip. Hold briefly.

2. V-pressure
Place your index finger and middle finger in a V above the child's lips. Push up and out. For the bottom lip, push down and out.

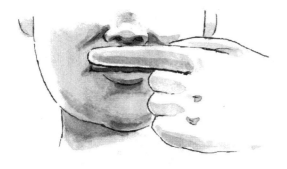

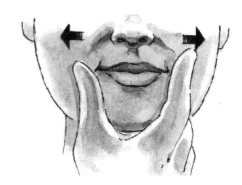

3. **mustache press**
   Place your index finger on the area
   above the child's top lip and press in.

4. **lip stroke**
   Place your thumb and index finger
   at the center of the child's lips.
   Stroke to corners and hold briefly.

Lip Rounding/Protruding Techniques

These techniques are important for /w, sh, ch/ and /j/ sounds.

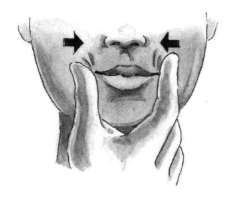

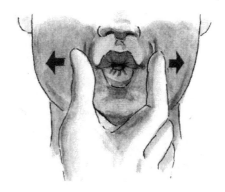

l. **pucker resistance**
   Have the child smile or say "ee"
   as you push his lips into a pucker.

2. **smile resistance**
   Have the child pucker or say "ooh"
   as you pull his lips into a smile.

109

Central Groove of the Tongue Techniques

These techniques are important for /s, z, sh, ch, j, er, r/ and /th/ sounds.

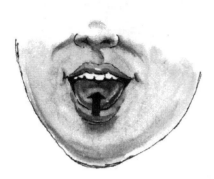
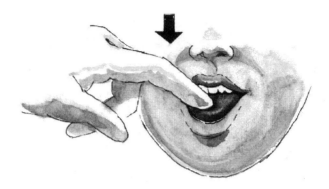

1. **central groove stroke**
   Stroke the central groove of the child's tongue from the tip to halfway back.

2. **central groove tap**
   Administer quick taps to the child's tongue along the central groove from the tip to halfway back.

Tongue Tip/Front Elevation and Spreading Techniques

These techniques are important for /t, d, n, l, s, z, sh, ch, j, er/ and /r/ sounds.

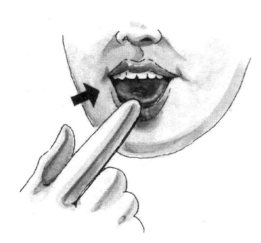
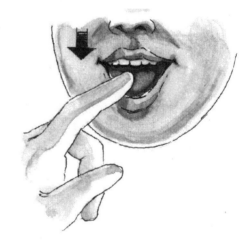

1. **tongue tip press: in**
   Press into the child's tongue tip. Repeat and have the child push back.

2. **tongue tip press: down**
   Push down on the child's tongue tip. Repeat and have the child push up.

110

Chapter 8
The Source for Down Syndrome

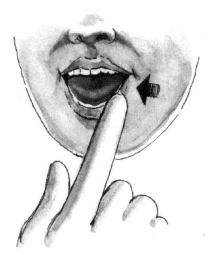

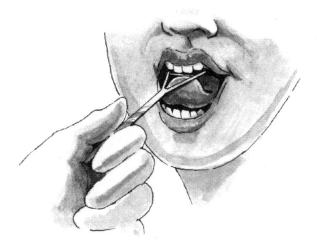

3. **tongue tip press: lateral**
   Push into each side of the child's
   tongue. Repeat and have the child
   push back.

4. **tongue tip elevation**
   Place a small dental floss holder
   with floss in it behind the child's
   front teeth. Have the child tap or
   sustain touch on the floss with his
   tongue tip.

Tongue Back Elevation Techniques

These techniques are important for /k, g, er, r/ and /y/ sounds.

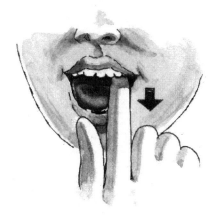

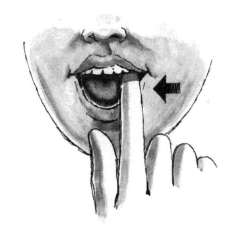

I. **tongue back press: top**
   Push down on the top back of each
   side of the child's tongue.

2. **tongue back press: sides**
   Push into the back sides of the
   child's tongue.

III

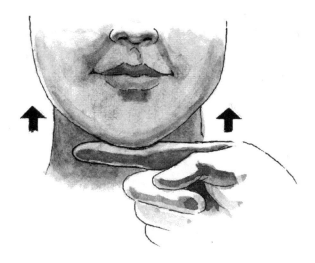

3. tongue base press
Push up on the base of the child's tongue by pressing upward behind the chin with your index finger.

Tongue Lateral Margin Elevation and Spreading Techniques

These techniques are important for /t, d, n, s, z, sh, ch, j, er, r, l/ and /y/ sounds.

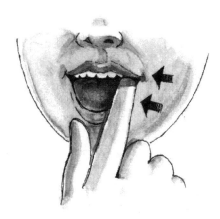

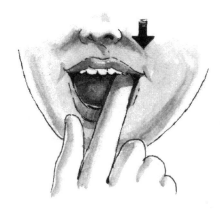

1. tongue side press: in
Put finger along the entire side of the child's tongue and push in toward the midline.

2. tongue side press: down
Put finger along the entire side of the top of the child's tongue and push down.

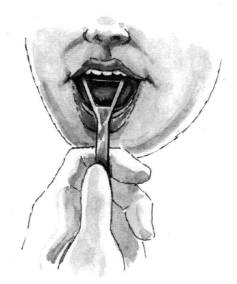

3. **tongue spread**
   Place a standard-size dental floss holder
   between the child's molars. Have the child
   spread his tongue so its sides touch the sides
   of the dental floss holder.

Tongue Retraction Techniques

These techniques are important for /k, g, y/ and /r/ sounds. You can also use the tongue tapping technique from the *Central Groove of the Tongue Techniques* on page 110 using deep pressure.

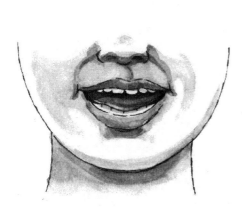

1. **tongue bite**
   Have the child gently bite on the sides
   of his tongue between his molars and
   slide his tongue back.

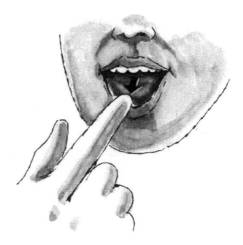

2. **tongue stroke**
   Stroke the child's tongue along the
   central groove from halfway back
   to the tongue tip.

Resistive Sucking

Sucking increases lip closure, lip strength, graded jaw closure and stability, and use of the cheek muscles.

Make sure the child holds the straw with her lips, not her teeth. Encourage a stronger suck by using straws of various widths or shapes or twisted aquarium tubing. Use thicker drinking substances for greater sucking strength. Partially freeze drinks in plastic bottles. Have the child put her lips around the bottle and suck.

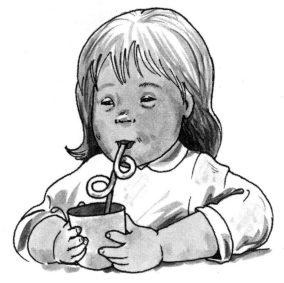

Sustained Blowing

Blowing facilitates lip closure and rounding, facial tone, graded jaw positioning and movements, and breath support for speech.

Gradiate the tasks by using blowing items or activities that require greater or lesser air flow, lip strength, lip contact, lip rounding, and jaw opening. Make sure the child holds the item for blowing with her lips, not her teeth. Use items such as:

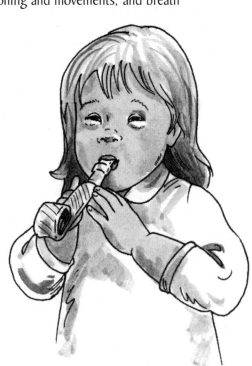

- blowing toys (any toy that primarily uses blowing like horns or whistles)
- beach balls (child blows it up)
- sound makers (harmonica, whistle)
- paper party blowers that roll up
- bubbles (wands, bubble pipes, straws, flexible tubing like aquarium tubing)
- small plastic balls (child blows them around with air directly from her mouth or by using a straw)
- straws of different widths and shapes
- two-liter bottles (child puts her lips around the top and blows into it)

Appendix B: Consonant Hand Signals

These hand signals can be used during speech practice to provide visual, kinesthetic, and/or tactile cues.

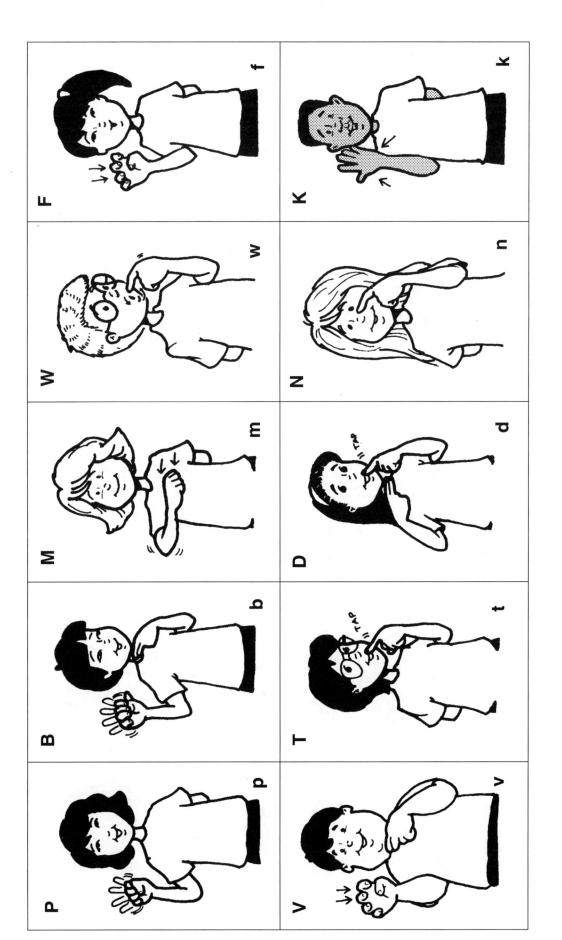

Chapter 8
The Source for Down Syndrome

Appendix B: Consonant Hand Signals, *continued*

These hand signals can be used during speech practice to provide visual, kinesthetic, and/or tactile cues.

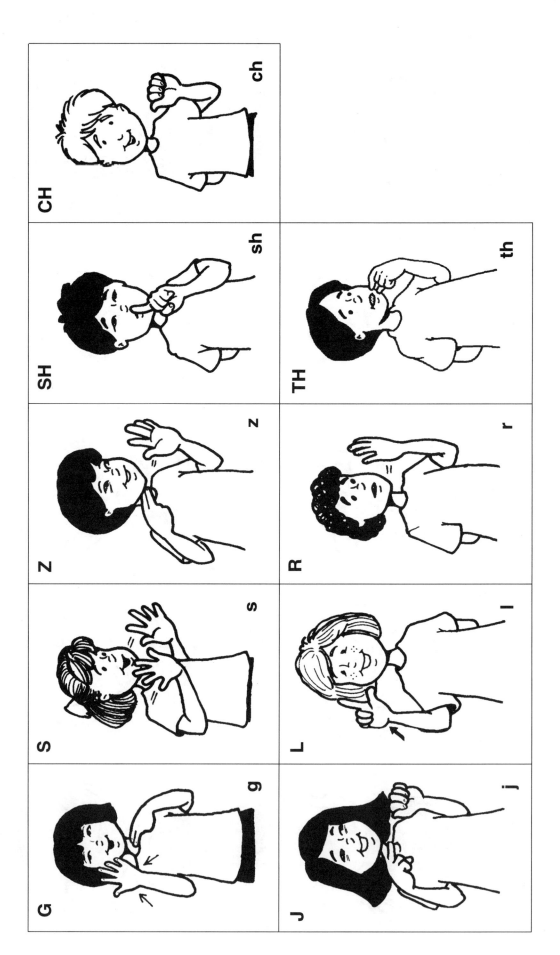

Consonant Hand Signal Descriptions

These hand signal descriptions are for the consonant signals pictured on pages 115 and 116.
Use whichever hand is more comfortable for you and your student.

p	Make fist at shoulder level, palm facing out. Open your fingers quickly as you say "p."
b	Same motion as "p," but put other hand on throat as you say "b."
m	Make a fist with palm down. Pull fist slowly across body at chest level as you say "m."
w	Use index finger to circle lips as you say "w."
f	Make claw, palm facing out at face level. Move hand down as you say "f."
v	Same motion as "f," but other hand is on throat.
t	Tap index finger on top lip as you say "t."
d	Same motion as "t," but put other hand on throat as you say "d."
n	Put index finger on nose as you say "n."
k	Open hand by shoulder, palm facing back. Move hand over shoulder as you say "k."
g	Same motion as "k," but put other hand on throat as you say "g."
s	Open both hands at chest level, with palms facing out. Push hands out as you say "s."
z	Similar motion as "s," but put one hand on throat as you say "z."
sh	Put your index finger on lips as you say "sh."
ch	Make fist at shoulder level, facing out. Push up fist as you say "ch."
j	Same motion as "ch," but put other hand on throat as you say "j."
l	Hold index finger and thumb in L-shape at mouth level, facing out as you say "l."
r	Open hand, palm facing you at mouth level. Move hand away from mouth as you say "r."
th	Use index finger and thumb to pretend to pull tongue between teeth as you say "th."

117

Chapter 9: Augmentative Communication

We all use strategies to augment our verbal communication. Infants start at an early age augmenting their attempts to communicate using smiles, eye gaze, and body movement. As adults we use gesture, facial expressions, and pointing to support our communication. We employ what we need to make our messages understood. We need to facilitate the use of natural and formal augmentative communication systems with the Down syndrome population to support and improve their ability to communicate.

Individuals with Down syndrome typically demonstrate higher receptive language skills than expressive skills. Their problems with oral communication make it difficult for the children to communicate effectively, which may lead to passivity, learned helplessness, and possible communication avoidance or challenging behaviors. The use of alternative or augmentative communication can help overcome a child's expressive inabilities, and enhance his ability to communicate with others and to act on his environment.

This chapter is not a review of all available types of augmentative, alternative, or assistive communication systems. Rather, this chapter will review the rationale for using augmentative communication with the Down syndrome population and the common types of augmentative devices and systems that have been used effectively. For most individuals with Down syndrome, augmentative communication is used to support communication and learning as they develop speech and expanded language skills. These individuals learn most effectively using a Total Communication approach which capitalizes on the strength of their visual skills.

Definition of Alternative or Augmentative Communication

Alternative or augmentative communication is the use of any device, technique, symbol system, or combination thereof to supplement, enhance, or increase a person's communication abilities. Augmentative communication provides support and an alternative way to communicate wants, needs, messages, and ideas. Using an augmentative device or system of communication can circumvent specific areas of disability, can support learning, and can facilitate communication.

The type of augmentative system(s) selected depends on the individual's level of cognitive, language, motor, and social skill development; presence of sensory deficits; specific learning and communication needs; and the type of response he is able to produce. There is a wide range of augmentative systems and devices available. They range from the use of natural gestures to electronic devices with speech synthesizers. There are devices and systems available for those who have severely limited cognitive and physical abilities. There are also devices and systems for those with near normal cognitive and receptive language skills, but who need support in communicating due to limited speech and expressive language skills.

An augmentative communication system can be specifically designed to communicate a single idea or request or be used as a multi-level and multi-functional system to assist an individual in all aspects of his life.

Why Augmentative Communication Is Used with the Down Syndrome Population

Individuals with Down syndrome demonstrate significant difficulty developing speech and expressive language skills. Use of augmentative communication is effective in teaching cognitive and language skills, as well as serving as a bridge to the development of effective expressive communication.

Advantages of Using Augmentative Communication

Advantages of using augmentative systems with the Down syndrome population include the following:

- allows the individual to interact with and control his environment
- circumvents the transient nature of spoken language and areas of weakness, including deficits in auditory perception and processing, speech, oral-motor skills, vision, and hearing
- validates and builds self-esteem and confidence as a communicator
- provides an accepted supplemental means of communication for those with limited speech and language abilities
- allows the child to communicate commensurate with his level of receptive language development and mental age
- helps develop the ability to communicate in a symbolic way
- provides a means to teach, practice, and produce words, word combinations, syntax, morphological structures (i.e., word endings), and pragmatic skills
- motivates the child to continue to develop communication skills
- clarifies the child's communication attempts and meanings
- reduces learned helplessness by providing an effective means for the individual to communicate wants, needs, and ideas

- reduces negative behaviors, frustration, and stress that may develop from the inability to communicate
- increases social interaction
- increases independence
- provides multi-sensory input using the stronger modalities
- is mutually reinforcing for both conversational partners
- increases attention skills
- increases others' perceptions and expectations of the individual's capabilities
- takes the child out of the passive respondent role to make him a more active communicator
- allows the child to express his emotions
- can be adapted over time to meet the individual's changing needs

Prerequisite Skills for the Use of Augmentative Communication Systems

There are specific prerequisite skills that should be in place before an individual can be successful using augmentative communication. These skills can vary with the form of augmentative communication system selected. Skills and areas of functioning to assess and consider when selecting a form(s) of augmentative communication should include the child's:

- level of awareness; ability to attend; use and maintain eye contact; and visual scanning ability
- ability to visually track objects and individuals
- ability to shift attention
- visual and auditory figure-ground skills (e.g., ability to attend to the parent's voice in the presence of background noise)
- development of looking, listening, reaching, and interest in his environment
- level of communicative intent and a need to communicate
- level of cognitive functioning (needs to be at Piaget's stage 6 level of sensorimotor development)
- joint attention and interaction skills
- ability to take conversational turns
- ability to make choices
- ability to imitate (This skill is helpful, but not required.)
- physical and motor capabilities

▸ ability to maintain postural position and head control

▸ ability to maintain position and range of movement of the arms, hands, and fingers

▸ motor coordination and control to select, point, exchange, or produce signs

- presence of sensory deficits
- visual and auditory processing strengths and weaknesses
- level of language comprehension
- present means of nonverbal and verbal communication and the strategies the child employs
- social and pragmatic skills
- adaptive and self-help skills
- consistency and readability of behavior

Selecting the Correct Form of Augmentative Communication

Each form or type of augmentative communication has specific user requirements and skills that must be in place or taught before the individual can be successful using it. Selection of a specific device or system will depend on the individual's cognitive, language, sensory, and motor skills; the type(s) of response he is able to make; demonstration of the prerequisite skills; his specific learning, communication, and daily living needs; and his level of motivation. The selection of the appropriate device or system is often a team decision, which includes the individual who will use the system, his parents, teachers, therapists, and other significant people in his life. The augmentative communication system should:

- improve communication skills immediately
- increase the desire to communicate
- increase the frequency of communication
- increase the opportunity and amount of participation in all activities
- be accepted by others
- be portable
- be affordable
- be adaptable for current and future communication needs
- be user-friendly
- be easily repaired
- be functional in all aspects of the individual's life

- be usable by all communication partners
- improve the level and complexity of communication

Types of Augmentative Communication Used with the Down Syndrome Population

Augmentative systems fall into two categories, aided or unaided, and use different symbol systems to produce a message. Augmentative communication systems typically used with the Down syndrome population include both aided and unaided systems in combination with verbalization in a Total Communication approach.

Aided Systems

An aided system displays the symbols or vocabulary on some form of equipment, platform, or device. Concrete symbols and abstract symbols can be used on an aided system including objects, a piece of or a miniature object, two-dimensional pictures, photographs, drawings, words, or abstract symbols (e.g., Blissymbols®). Devices include language boards, communication books, computers, and switch-activated or electronic communication systems. These devices use direct selection (e.g., pointing, touching) which is the simplest and fastest form of selection and the type most often used by the Down syndrome population.

The advantages of using an aided communication system with the Down syndrome population include the following:

- requires lower level of motor skill and complexity of movement to select symbols and produce a message
- validates the individual as a communicator
- can build self-esteem
- motivates the individual to continue to develop communication skills
- uses highly salient words for communication
- most are user-friendly (i.e., easy to learn and understand)
- adapts to a wide range of handicapping conditions
- allows the individual to generate language at a higher level than he may presently be able to verbalize
- allows a combination of symbols to produce phrases and sentences

- easy to obtain, program, make, or reproduce (i.e., make more than one copy)
- message is easily interpreted by the communication partner

The disadvantages of using an aided communication system with the Down syndrome population include the following:

- needs training to use
- less portable
- may be expensive
- has limited flexibility as far as the vocabulary used and the messages that can be formulated
- requires monitoring (e.g., batteries)
- can be broken or lost
- may need to be serviced (e.g., upgrade, repair), which can leave the user without a communication system

Unaided Systems

Unaided systems require nothing more than the individual's body to communicate an idea, request, or comment. Common unaided systems effectively used by the Down syndrome population include use of manual sign, gestures, and facial expressions.

The advantages of using an unaided communication system with the Down syndrome population includes the following:

- portability
- no equipment needed (signs and gestures are easily produced)
- signs can be adapted to meet the individual's needs
- new vocabulary can be introduced spontaneously to meet individual, activity, or situation needs
- low cost, no servicing required
- does not require batteries or electricity

The disadvantages of using an unaided communication system with the Down syndrome population includes the following:

- not as easily understood by others without specific training

- requires higher-level motor planning and motor skills than aided devices
- messages require a listener to be present, plus there is no way to store or leave a message
- may not be functional for individuals with severe handicaps
- the complexity of the message is often lower than the individual's receptive abilities (i.e., higher-level morphological structures are not often expressed in the signs or gestures)
- the individual must generate a message or response without the support of pictures or written words

Intervention

There are many forms of augmentative communication that can be used to assist the individual with Down syndrome develop and improve his communication skills.

1. Object Selection: The child chooses between two or more objects presented to express his basic wants and needs. Objects may be displayed on a board, placed in a basket, or placed on the table for direct selection (e.g., a cup and a spoon; the child can select the cup to request a drink and the spoon to request another bite of food).

2. Picture Selection or Exchange: Same as object selection, but uses pictures, line drawings, or photographs to indicate wants or needs. For picture exchange, the child must give the picture to another individual to indicate his choice, want, or need.

3. Choice Box: Usually includes a larger variety of objects to select from (three or more). The child selects the object that represents what he wants (e.g., cup for drink). Real objects, miniatures, or pictures may be used to represent the child's choices (e.g., toys, foods, clothes, activities, and places the child wants to go).

4. Language Board: Uses a selected core of concrete or abstract symbols or a combination of the two including pictures, line drawings, or photographs specifically arranged on a board or computer to help the child communicate with others.

5. Communication Books: Uses pictures, drawings, photographs, objects, and pieces of objects to communicate wants, needs, and comments; to clarify; and to respond to others. These books may be arranged by or incorporate a specific subject matter (e.g., My Friends, Safety Words and Signs, Food).

6. Classroom Dictionary: Uses pictures, drawings, or photographs and incorporates vocabulary, concepts, phrases and sentences needed for classroom success.

7. Gesture Modes: Uses body language, facial expression, fine motor and gross motor movements to communicate. Gesture is a natural developmental process in all children and adults and is used to assist or enhance their verbal communication. The universal use and acceptance of gesture makes it easy to learn and understand.

8. Manual Sign: There are several different forms of manual sign which differ in complexity. The type of manual sign selected will depend on the child's cognitive and language levels and his sensory and motor skills.

Use of manual sign with the Down syndrome population is usually very effective because of their strong visual and gestural skills. The use of manual sign to support and augment communication attempts should begin when the child is an infant. Children with Down syndrome can learn signs as early as 12 months. They typically use manual sign until around the age of five, when they stop depending on the signs and become predominantly verbal communicators.

9. Switch-activated Communication Devices: Switches can be used to enhance learning and communication for a wide range of individuals with handicaps. Switches can be used to activate a toy or device, to request, or to make a choice.

10. Electronic Communication Devices: These are systems programmed to facilitate communication and learning. Most are commercially produced (e.g., computers) and are adapted for specific user needs.

Suggested Developmental Progression for Teaching Sign (Klein, 1988)

- Start by using gross gestures before introducing signs and words (e.g., pat chair for *sit*, motion with arm for *come here*, wave *bye*).
- Start with signs that are motorically and developmentally the easiest to produce (e.g., *eat*).
- Use highly salient words.
- Teach signs that incorporate touch (e.g., *my, mother*).
- Teach signs that utilize hand and arm movements toward the body, then away from the body (e.g., *come, go*).
- Teach signs produced with the hands coming together (e.g., *more*).
- Teach signs that use one hand, then two hands (e.g., *drink, in*).
- Teach signs that have one hand dominant or used to assist the other hand (e.g., *on*).
- Teach two hands doing opposite movements (e.g., *walk, car*).

11. Total Communication: This pairs simultaneous production of speech and manual sign or another augmentative device or symbol system (e.g., pictures or pictures and print). It is a multi-component communication system.

Total Communication

Total Communication is generally the most successful form of augmentative communication to promote development of learning and communication in the Down syndrome population. Use of Total Communication promotes expressive language skills as well as speech skills. It is often described as a "transitional mode of communication" for the Down syndrome child. This is because the child typically replaces his use of an augmentative communication system with oral communication around his fifth or sixth birthday. The use of Total Communication may be continued after the child has become a verbal communicator to provide multi-sensory support for learning and expansion of expressive morpho-syntactic skills.

Types of augmentative communication most often used in a Total Communication approach with the Down syndrome population include verbalization and one or more of the following:

- gesture
- objects
- pictures and/or picture symbols
- abstract symbols
- communication boards
- manual sign
- pictures plus printed words
- printed words
- switch-activated device
- electronic device

Advantages of using Total Communication with the Down syndrome population include the following:

- promotes, enhances, and supports communication and learning
- capitalizes on areas of strength for the individual with Down syndrome which include use of gesture, receptive language, pragmatics, social skills, visual perception, and early literacy skills
- increases interaction between speaker and listener
- provides multi-sensory cues
- increases the overall size of vocabulary because the child with Down syndrome tends to learn a different set of words in sign than he uses verbally
- promotes speech, does not inhibit it
- may reduce the extent of the early language delay by providing a functional mode of communication
- provides more opportunities to communicate
- serves as a transitional communication system to oral communication
- increases attending skills
- may diminish learned helplessness and development of challenging behaviors by providing a way to act on and control the environment
- is functional in most settings
- most forms are universally accepted and can serve to facilitate understanding by and integration with peers
- most forms of augmentative communication can be adapted to be used with the Down syndrome population
- allows the individual to produce and rehearse words, phrases, sentences, and morpho-syntactic structures (e.g., use of plural /s/, past tense /ed/) that he is unable to currently generate on his own
- more tangible than just the spoken word

When introducing and teaching an augmentative communication system to a child, it is important that:

- the child demonstrates the necessary prerequisite skills to use augmentative communication
- the child's communication needs have been determined
- the type(s) of augmentative communication selected is/are developmentally appropriate
- it is as user-friendly as possible
- the augmentative system is functional and will immediately enhance and increase the child's communication attempts
- the system is treated as a valid communication system by the child, parents, siblings, teachers, and peers
- the communication partner also uses the system to communicate during daily activities, action routines, and scripts
- it is accessible and portable for the individual
- the system can be updated or repaired in a timely manner
- the child can be taught the vocabulary that is used on the system
- the symbols used are understood by all communication partners

Principles to follow when introducing Total Communication or augmentative communication:

1. Make sure the child is attending.

2. Make sure the child has something to communicate.

3. Select a core vocabulary and introduce it one item at a time. Use a variety of words including objects, people, places, actions, concepts, and feelings.

4. Incorporate pragmatic functions when teaching vocabulary.

5. Use symbols that are universally understood.

6. Use error-free learning by breaking instruction into small steps.

7. Pair presentation (e.g., picture symbol/sign) simultaneously with speech.

8. Be consistent in presentation, model, and cues.

9. When introducing the augmentative system, use play and engaging activities to get the child to respond.

10. If the child is using a device, let him explore it on his own to become familiar with it.

11. Provide all the necessary cues and prompts for the child to be successful.

12. Provide the child with lots of practice and drill in daily home, therapy, and classroom activities.

13. Reward the child for using the system.

14. Make sure people significant to the child know how to use the system and use it consistently.

15. Adults, siblings, and peers should use the device or system to communicate during daily, classroom, and therapy activities and during play.

16. Teach vocabulary sets in real activities and practice them in daily routines as well as incorporate them into classroom activities; then expand to scripted activities. Keep the vocabulary current.

17. Set up situations to encourage the child to practice and use the system.

18. Use pictures, picture symbols, and print to facilitate attention, learning, transitions, and independence both at home and in the classroom. Some situations where it may be helpful are:

    - daily schedules and reminders
    - to label materials in the classroom or clothing drawers at home
    - work and job charts
    - vocabulary theme books
    - scripts
    - storyboards

19. Adapt the system as needed for the child to be successful.

20. Establish a way for all users to comment on usefulness and any need for change.

21. Be adaptable and flexible (e.g., if the child has visual handicaps, use large print or black-line pictures; if the child is unable to make a conventional sign, adapt it to his ability; if the child has a hearing loss, use visual cues in the classroom to signal him to attend to the teacher).

22. Don't ask too many questions. The child needs to initiate and use the system to communicate, not just to respond.

Chapter 10: Voice, Resonance, and Fluency Issues

Voice and Resonance

Individuals with Down syndrome often present voice and/or resonance problems which can affect speech intelligibility. The voice in an individual with Down syndrome is often described as hoarse or husky, harsh, gruff, breathy, gutteral, low-pitched, and/or monotonous. The person with Down syndrome may exhibit hyponasal or hypernasal resonance or excessive nasal emission of air on consonant productions with the presence of nasal snorts or fricatives.

Generally there is a similar fundamental frequency in typically-developing children and in children with Down syndrome in the later elementary school years and during adolescence. There does not appear to be a pattern of restricted fundamental frequency range. Consequently, fundamental frequency does not require intervention in voice therapy with the child or adolescent with Down syndrome.

There is an increase in frequency perturbations (i.e., irregularities in vocal fold vibration cycles) which may be related to perceived hoarseness in some individuals with Down syndrome. Amplitude perturbations tend to be irregular in those with voice disorders. Perceptually these are perceived as a rough or harsh vocal quality.

A major contributor to voice problems in people with Down syndrome is a reduction in muscle tone. This results in a weakened vocal mechanism which may have difficulty maintaining a consistent amount of vocal fold tension. There may be air loss at the level of the vocal folds due to incomplete sealing which can result in breathiness, harshness, or decreased volume. Greater levels of energy may be required to activate vocal fold vibrations. This flaccidity in the laryngeal muscles may result in a hoarse, harsh, or gruff voice quality.

In addition, low tone in the respiratory system may make it difficult to produce and sustain a consistent air supply for speech. This consistent air supply with somewhat steady pressure is necessary for the vocal folds to open and close in a smooth pattern. A lack of air supply can also affect loudness levels.

The usual pattern of loudness found in individuals with Down syndrome is decreased volume. It may be due to hypotonia, irregular vocal fold closing for air buildup, decreased breath support for loudness, and/or a history of hearing loss. It's possible that some of the language production patterns characteristic in Down syndrome speech, including the use of shorter utterances and less complex syntax, may be influenced by voice disorders. The individual may not be able to produce voice long enough to sustain longer and more complex sentences.

It is common to find a pattern of allergies and increased incidence of upper respiratory infection in individuals with Down syndrome. These can contribute to a hoarse, breathy, or harsh vocal quality as well as hyponasal resonance.

127

Resonance refers to the tonal quality of speech. Hyponasal resonance may be found in the individual with Down syndrome secondary to septum deviations, small nasal openings and sinuses, enlarged tonsils and adenoids, allergies, and a pattern of upper respiratory infection. These conditions call for medical, rather than speech therapy, because voice therapy will not change the hyponasal pattern.

Individuals with Down syndrome tend to have a greater degree and severity of hypernasality than their typically-developing peers. It may be manifested by touch closure (i.e., where the velum barely touches the pharyngeal walls to close off the nasopharynx for production of non-nasal speech sounds) of the velopharyngeal mechanism which typically is displayed in speech as nasal "snorts" and nasal fricatives on consonant productions or in hypernasality on vowel productions. Velopharyngeal incompetence can be secondary to a short velum, flaccid muscles in the velopharyngeal mechanism, difficulty with velopharyngeal closure, and/or a smaller oral cavity with a large tongue which may force more air nasally. Some children have an intact velopharyngeal mechanism but have excessive nasal emission of air because of difficulty with the timing of palatal movements or coordinating of these movements. They also may have difficulties with jaw stability and placement during speech that can affect palatal movement.

Individuals with Down syndrome may make their already present voice problems worse through vocal abuse and misuse. They tend to engage in vocally abusive behaviors such as intermittent loud speaking volume, sudden and hard phonational onsets, and frequent yelling. In these cases, it is important to implement a vocal hygiene program.

Intervention

1. Medical treatment may be recommended for some voice or resonance disorders.

    a. Hyponasality – Inspection of the nasal passages, nasal septum, sinuses, tonsils, or adenoids is necessary to determine the cause of the air blockage. Surgery or other medical intervention may be warranted if there is a significant problem in one or more of these areas. The presence of allergies should be determined and treated as needed.

    b. Hypernasality – The velopharyngeal mechanism should be inspected for a short palate, a submucous cleft palate, or velopharyngeal incompetence. If the hypernasality does not respond to speech therapy, a palatal lift may be helpful if the child can tolerate it, or a pharyngeal flap may be needed.

        Adenoid removal may result in hypernasality if the adenoid pad was used to aid in velopharyngeal closure. It may be beneficial to do videofluoroscopy to determine palatal and pharyngeal functioning and relationships before an adenoidectomy is performed. A lateral adenoidectomy can leave the bulk of the tissue intact for palatal contact, while removing the portion that may impede on the Eustachian tube or impact breathing.

    c. Hoarseness, harshness, or breathiness – The nasopharynx and vocal folds should be inspected by an Ear, Nose, and Throat physician for abnormalities such as swelling, redness, thickening, or polyps or nodules on the vocal folds. If allergies impact the vocal mechanism, they should be treated.

2. Speech therapy may be recommended for some voice or resonance disorders.

    a. Hypernasality and excessive nasal emission of nasal air

        -   develop good foundations for appropriate resonance such as appropriate body positioning, jaw stability and grading, and appropriate articulator placements for consonant productions

        -   slow the rate, pause slightly between words or phrases, and incorporate other prosody work in order to give the velopharyngeal mechanism time to make and coordinate adjustments during speech

- practice producing a series of non-nasal/ nasal sustained phonemes (e.g., "ahhhmmmmmmmmmahhh")

- use a larger mouth opening during speech (i.e, overarticulate at the front of the mouth to facilitate increased movements of the muscles at the back of the mouth)

- reduce sound duration and air pressure on strident productions

- do blowing activities as a means to facilitate knowledge and monitoring of oral airflow

- facilitate muscle tone throughout the body, face, and speech mechanism with movement and touch-input activities (e.g., positioning the child, face pats)

- individuals with hypernasality secondary to timing problems may benefit from an apraxia-type program that concentrates on gradually learning to make articulatory shifts while slowly building performance load (e.g., building from production of syllables to words to multisyllabic words to phrases and then to sentences)

b. Hoarseness or harshness – Use techniques to decrease vocal abuse and misuse if these are contributing causes to the hoarse or harsh voice quality (i.e., learning the types and causes of vocal abuse and misuse and developing more appropriate vocal behaviors)

Vocal abuse and misuse behaviors include the following:

- inappropriate voice volume and pitch
- talking over noise
- hard onset of speech
- yelling
- screaming
- loud talking or crying
- using animal or puppet voices
- making vehicle or environmental sounds

- excessive talking
- talking with too much force
- frequent throat clearing or coughing

Appropriate vocal behaviors include the following:

- getting the listener's attention in ways other than yelling or calling loudly (e.g., walking over to the listener)

- moving away from noisy environments before attempting conversation

- standing closer to the listener in noisy environments

- using pom-poms, signs, or clapping instead of yelling at sports events

- reducing amounts of talking

- reducing periods of loud crying

- increasing intake of water

- treating allergies to reduce throat clearing and coughing

- using an easy onset of voice

- using periods of vocal rest

c. Low volume – Voice volume can be increased by facilitating more normal muscle tone. This can be done through movement (i.e., gross motor activities) and appropriate body positioning with the back upright rather than slumped. Breath control and support for speech can be targeted through movement and blowing activities. Be careful not to use activities to increase volume that would cause a further strain on the voice (e.g., talking over noise, using too much force in attempts to increase volume).

d. Breathiness – Breathiness may be decreased by facilitating appropriate muscle tone in the abdominal area and by strengthening the adductor muscles of the larynx. Working on breath support for speech may facilitate a more normal vocal quality.

e. Monotonous voice – Prosody work can help establish appropriate intonational contours, syllable and word stress, speaking rate, and separation between words in sentences.

Fluency

Some individuals with Down syndrome demonstrate disfluent speech or stuttering, particularly higher functioning and more verbal individuals. Disfluent speech or stuttering may be secondary to:

- neurologic or physiologic factors
- hypotonicity
- motor planning and coordination difficulties
- auditory memory and processing difficulties
- inefficient breath support for speech
- language disorders
- formulation difficulties
- latency of response
- prosody and rate disturbances
- phonological disorders

Intervention

Selection of intervention goals and techniques will depend on the severity of the child's stuttering and the types of characteristics present in her speech. Intervention areas may include the following:

1. Consult with the parents to gather their concerns and expectations for their child, the degree and type of stuttering noted, when the stuttering began, the consistency of the stuttering, the presence of secondary characteristics, strategies that have been employed, health problems, the child's typical daily schedule, and pressures the child may be facing.

   Educate the parents about disfluency and stuttering, definitions, etiology, characteristics, and ranges of severity.

Teach the parents how to be good speech models by using a slowed rate of speech and simplified language, giving the child eye contact during conversations, and letting the child finish her message before responding.

Have the parents keep a daily fluency diary that documents the child's periods of fluency and dysfluency and the situations or pressures associated with them.

Counsel the parents to reduce communicative stress for the child by:

- reducing performance demands

- reducing the number of questions asked

- not calling attention to the stuttering

- validating the child's communicative messages by putting more emphasis on the content of the message rather than the way it was delivered

- allowing the child more time to process and then formulate a response

- reducing interruptions and distractions as well as not interrupting the child

- not talking at the same time as the child (overtalking)

Teach the parents simple strategies to encourage more fluent speech by having them:

- encourage the child to use a slower rate of speech (e.g., using a signal to remind the child to slow her rate, having adults use a slower rate of speech, slowing down the child's daily schedule and pace of activities)

- encourage the child to take her time to formulate and deliver a message or response by waiting and giving the child attention and eye contact

The Source for Down Syndrome

- encourage the child to wait until her conversational partner has finished talking before beginning a response

- encourage the child to use an easy onset to her speech

2. Assess the child's fluency, language, and speech skills; processing and memory skills; oral-motor skills, breath support for speech; and hearing. Plan intervention to address specific areas of weakness.

3. Educate the child about her dysfluency in terms she can understand.

4. Help the child develop appropriate respiration and breath support for speech by:

- facilitating correct posture and positioning that encourages trunk stability

- facilitating general muscle tone and strength of the abdominal muscles

- doing sustained blowing activities

- producing sustained vowel productions

- teaching the child to use shorter utterance, to not speak on residual air, and to monitor when her air is running out during speech

5. Teach the child rate control by:

- modeling and practicing the use of a slower rate of speech; have adults around the child do the same

- using a pacing board

- using rhythm or a beat as a pattern for speech rate

- incorporating prosody work such as developing intonation contours and appropriate stress on words in sentences to slow down the speaking rate

6. Teach the child to use an easy onset of speech by:

- using reduced pressure to initiate speech

- using relaxed productions

- using smoother onsets when initiating speech

  ▸ begin drill using syllables with initial /h/ to facilitate easy onset

  ▸ expand to one syllable, then multisyllabic real and nonsense initial /h/ words

  ▸ practice words that begin with vowels; add initial /h/ as needed to facilitate easy onset, gradually fading the use of /h/

  ▸ practice words that begin with consonants using light pressure between articulator contact points (e.g., have the child touch her lips together lightly when saying bilabial words)

- reinforcing the child when she uses "easy talking"

7. Teach the child to reduce her effort, struggle, and muscle tension by preparing the system for speech practice through activities to normalize tone, facilitate respiration/phonation, normalize oral-motor skills and planning, and to modulate alertness and awareness.

- use relaxation techniques to relax the muscles used for speech

- use positive mental imagery and positive self-talk

- use easy onset techniques

- use light pressure of articulatory contacts

8. Build oral-motor coordination and sequencing ability. Difficulty in this area appears to be a significant contributor to disfluency and stuttering in the Down syndrome population. An apraxia-type approach with emphasis on syllable productions and

performance loading is often effective (See Chapter 8, pages 92–93).

9. Build pragmatic skills. Teach the child to:

   • listen to the whole message from others before responding

   • appropriately take turns in a conversation (i.e., don't overtalk or interrupt conversational partners)

   • take time to process information, requests, or questions

   • take time to formulate responses

   • make conversational repairs and ask for clarifications as needed

10. Build times of fluency. Make the child aware of these times by using speaking to rhythm; using nursery rhymes, short utterances, and familiar utterances that can be produced with fluency; and pointing out the child's fluent productions.

Milestones for the Typically-Developing Child

Human development is a complex, genetically predetermined, pre-programmed process of growing and learning. Development occurs in a relatively specific sequence, with earlier skills providing foundations for later acquired skills which are consolidated and generalized over time. The development and learning process is affected by genetic, biological, psychological, cultural, and environmental factors. The typically-developing infant is born with neuromotor, attentional and perceptual abilities as well as the motivation to learn and communicate. All areas of development are interrelated and should be viewed as a whole. Growth in one area may affect growth in another area. Growth and development can't be controlled, but they can be influenced by many factors, including experience and the environment.

This section presents developmental scales for typically-developing children in the areas of:

- cognitive and play development
- gross and fine motor development
- oral-motor and feeding skills development
- speech development
- language development

The age levels are approximate and will vary with each child; consequently, these scales should be used as a general guideline.

Knowledge of typical development in all domains is important to understand the strengths and weaknesses of the child with Down syndrome. The child's genetics have a significant impact on his cognitive, biological, sensorimotor, communication, and psychological development. This knowledge is also needed when planning developmentally appropriate intervention.

Cognitive and Play Development

0 – 6 months

sees world as an extension of himself/herself
uses eye contact
knows environment will respond to needs
learns trust
explores and manipulates own body
will grasp object when placed in hand
begins to reach
visually tracks objects
puts objects in mouth
plays actively when propped up
shakes rattle
smiles when sees familiar face or toy
touches image in mirror
becomes excited when shown toy
tries to get toy out of reach
transfers toy from one hand to other
beginning of social interaction

6 – 12 months

grasps dangling object
uses fingers and mouth to explore toys
imitates simple movements
squeezes toys to make them squeak
likes to drop objects to watch them fall
performs differentiated actions with different objects
puts objects in and takes them out
uncovers hidden toy (object permanence)
acts on environment for specific purpose
   (i.e., cause and effect)
starts to demonstrate new actions on objects
puts rings on pegs
holds one object momentarily above another
pulls string to get toys (tool use)
plays "Peek-a-boo" and "Patty-cake"
begins functional play
uses different motor schemes for different toys
   (e.g., hugs a stuffed dog, shakes a rattle)

1.0 – 1.5 years (12 – 18 months)

demonstrates knowledge of means-end, causality,
   object permanence, and expanded tool use

explores and manipulates objects by inserting, pulling,
   emptying, and filling containers
plays alone for short periods of time
uses a variety of motor schemes in play
shows and/or offers objects to others
constructive play begins
explores toys to identify the parts responsible for their
   operation
scribbles spontaneously with crayon
likes to pick up objects and throw things
imitates daily household activities
demonstrates rapid shifts in attention
begins to symbolize

1.5 – 2.0 years (18 – 24 months)

demonstrates appropriate toy use
representational play begins
gives objects to adult to operate
demonstrates adult routines in play
object permanence is fully developed
representational imitation occurs (delayed or deferred
   imitation present)
begins to match like objects
likes games such as "Peek-a-Boo" and "Chase and
   Capture" (i.e., "I'm gonna get you!")
can arrange objects by size
knows multiple uses and ways to play with a toy
explores objects fully
demonstrates parallel play
talks to self in play
strings beads
enjoys playing with clay and Play-Doh®
uses objects as tools
relates action to an object or person
combines two toys in play
fits related objects together
presents fewer rapid attention shifts
extends symbolic play to include others
understands state and simple locative relations
   (e.g., *Mama happy, shoe on*)

2.0 – 3.0 years	3.0 – 4.0 years
demonstrates more complex, creative, and constructive play behaviors; exploration is now integrated with other types of play	has cognitive base for past and future tense
	prefers to play in small groups
stacks up to six blocks to knock down	begins to organize toys in an imaginative way
parallel play most common	assigns dolls personalities and plays with them as would a real friend
dependent on realistic props in play	
pretends actions of others	enjoys playing dress-up
some limited short sequences of action in a play scheme (e.g., puts doll's pajamas on, places in bed, covers up, gives doll a teddy bear, signals others to be quiet)	uses a related sequence of pretend events (e.g., picks up purse, gets keys out, pretends to get in a car made from two chairs, drives to store)
	demonstrates more associative play with others, but not fully cooperative
enjoys sand and water play (e.g., pour, dump, fill)	play does not require realistic props
matches objects by single dimension (e.g., puts all shoes together, sorts blocks from beads)	uses one object to represent another in play
	does not have to have previous experience with an activity to incorporate it into play
begins real interactive play with peers	builds structures and names them
re-enacts previous events with new outcomes	interested in exploring new places
dramatic play emerges	hypothesizes about future
thought is no longer tied to concrete objects	puts toys away on request
can make associations	doll and puppet play becomes more elaborate
arranges toys into meaningful groups	dramatic play increases along with the use of imaginary characters
puts three blocks in a row to make a train	
more associative play with others, but not cooperative play	comprehends textures (e.g., wet, rough, bumpy)
	enjoys playing "Hide-and-Seek"
can reason and remember	
anticipates consequences	**4.0 – 5.0 years**
builds with blocks, paints, completes puzzles, plays with clay	
pleased with attempts at art activity	continues to think concretely
dramatization and imagination used in play	shows off in dramatic play
takes a role during play, but roles change quickly	enjoys exploring a range of experiences, interests, and places
demonstrates symbolic play	plans play sequences in advance
begins to wait turn in play	begins to criticize own work
puts toys away with minimal help	wants more props in play, but no longer dependent on realistic props; uses imagination
can stack rings in order of size	
participates in stories and rhymes	starts to enjoy board games
begins to use abstraction	demonstrates early decision-making
can problem-solve using observation and reasoning	likes to work on projects and finish projects
performs action series (e.g., fills cup with sand, pours sand from cup onto plate, offers plate to friend)	can coordinate more than one event at a time
	enjoys playing in larger groups
can remember absent objects and events	enjoys competition and rivalry
recognizes colors	cooperative in play
applies previous experience to new problems	

135

Cognitive and Play Development, *continued*

5.0 – 6.0 years

plans out pretend situations in advance
can organize what will be needed in play
no longer depends on realistic props in play
may be interested in collecting items
plays games with rules
comprehends weight (e.g., understands that things can
    be heavy; knows that one object is heavier than
    another)

6.0 – 7.0 years

demonstrates a preoccupation for specific toys or
    objects
identifies specific qualities about self
develops from concrete to more abstract thought
    processes
demands more elaborate explanations
is egocentric
develops math and reading skills
memorizes information

2.0 – 4.0 Years: Piaget's Pre-operational Stage

During the pre-operational stage, the typically-developing child progresses from functioning primarily in a sensorimotor mode to a symbolic mode. The most important symbolic skill developed at this stage is the development of language. By 7 years of age, the child should have mastered skills such as multiple classification; class inclusion; and conservation of substance, weight, distance, and space.

7.0 – 11.0 Years: Piaget's Concrete Operations

At this stage, the child uses logical thought to solve concrete problems, rather than relying on his perceptions. He/she uses these thought processes to solve concrete problems including an understanding of transformations, using reversibility of thought, and mentally arranging objects by size. A portion of children with Down syndrome will accomplish skills at this level.

11.0 – 14.0 Years: Piaget's Formal Operations

By 11 years of age, the typically-developing child will have mastered Piaget's Concrete Operations stage and begun the formal operations stage of development. Beyond 11 years and by 14 years, the typically-developing child should have mastered Piaget's Formal Operations stage of development including skills such as thinking as an adult to solve problems, reasoning, and arriving at solutions.

                                               Milestones for the Typically-Developing Child
The Source for Down Syndrome

Gross motor skills pertain to those motor skills that allow the body to move through the environment including large movements of the arms, legs, and body. The following skills lay foundations for development in other areas.

Gross Motor Development	

0 – 6 months
 	
holds head up
focuses on learning to use his/her body
puts fist in mouth
develops control of arms and legs
reflexes present:
  • tonic neck reflex
  • rooting reflex
  • sucking reflex
  • startle or moro reflex
  • palmar or grasp reflex
  • plantar reflex
sits with support, head held steady, then sits unsupported
holds self erect when pulled to sitting position
progresses from random physical movement based on reflex to purposeful action
lifts head and chest when on stomach
begins to turn from tummy to back
reaches for objects in view
can grasp a rattle or toy
turns from side to side
hands engaged at mid-line (i.e., The child uses both hands together at the center of his/her body to do something like play with a toy or hold a bottle.)
	pulls self up to stand, holds on to furniture
	takes side steps while holding on
	moves from sitting to prone
	takes steps while adult holds hand
	bangs large objects
	attempts to throw objects
	takes first independent steps
	primitive reflexes gone
	demonstrates good head control

	1.0 – 1.5 years (12-18 months) goes from crawling to walking throws and rolls a ball climbs up stairs with help climbs onto chair walks as pushes a toy walks while carrying a toy or doll begins walking alone can open a closed door removes socks and shoes
6 – 12 months sits alone unsupported gains control of trunk rolls from back to stomach stands with support, then stands alone grasps scrunches knees under tummy prior to creeping moves to all fours position, starts to creep begins crawling pushes from stomach to sitting	**1.5 – 2.0 years (18 – 24 months)** begins with a wide stance, transitions to walking in adult manner climbs stairs, both feet on one step, independently goes down stairs with support walks backward kicks and throws ball sits self in chair jumps from bottom step begins to run and jump stands on one foot rides a mobility toy

137

2.0 – 2.5 years	4.0 – 6.0 years
kicks a ball briefly balances on one foot starts and stops running with ease takes a toy apart eats with spoon or fork climbs on furniture	dances balances on one foot 4-5 seconds skips using alternate feet runs on tiptoes climbs a ladder dresses self turns somersaults completes a broad jump marches in time to music follows the leader walks backward heel to toe jumps over a 8-10" high object runs with few falls while playing hops on either foot plays games

2.5 – 3.0 years	
stands on tiptoes jumps down off a step using both feet catches a large ball with straight arms begins to pedal a tricycle hops on one foot has mastered most of elementary motor skills 　(e.g., walking, standing, running, jumping)	

	6.0 – 12.0 years
3.0 – 4.0 years	develops ball-handling skills (e.g., throwing, bouncing, 　dribbling, catching, kicking) whistles learns to roller skate blows bubbles with bubble gum learns to swim stands on one foot for approximately 8 seconds learns to tie shoes sits for longer periods of time rides bicycle

3.0 – 4.0 years	
catches a large ball with arms bent walks on tiptoes walks heel to toe rides a tricycle, can turn corners walks a line for 10 feet swings on a swing sits with feet crossed at ankles alternates feet going down steps hops on one foot	

Fine motor skills are responsible for the control of smaller, more precise movements of the hands, fingers, eyes, face, and articulators.

Fine Motor Development	
0 – 6 months	**2.0 – 3.0 years**
clenches and opens fist looks at hands brings hands across mid-line (i.e., will take right hand and go across the body to grasp something on the left side of the body) grasp reflex disappears plays with hands, feet, toys, and clothing hands come together in play thumb does not participate in grasping objects grasp is limited to large objects approach to object is two-handed uses hand to reach, grasp, crumble, bang, and splash	takes toy apart uses spoon or fork fits toys together/snaps blocks together imitates a vertical and horizontal stroke imitates a continuous circle stroke imitates a zig-zag stroke begins to hold writing instrument more appropriately puts together a three-piece puzzle unscrews lid turns book pages singly starts to cut with scissors colors and starts to draw builds tower with up to six blocks strings beads pounds peg through a board snips paper when held by another person works latches and hooks good hand and finger coordination closes fist and moves thumb
6 – 12 months	
transfers object from one hand to the other hand holds rattle when placed in hand begins to release objects deliberately uses one-hand approach to grasping explores parts of a toy picks up small object using finger-thumb or pincer grasp puts object in a container one hand helps the other points with index finger	**3.0 – 4.0 years**
1.0 – 2.0 years (12 – 24 months)	develops preference for handedness uses scissors to cut across strip of paper while holding it assembles toys with more pieces completes puzzles with 5-15 pieces builds a 6-8 cube tower builds a three-block bridge from imitation draws simple figures puts on shoes initiates drawing a circle and a cross attempts to draw a person, details not complete makes things with clay paints with a brush or fingerpaints touches thumb to 2-4 fingers on same hand draws a recognizable object
puts rings on a stick or pegs in a peg board turns 2-3 book pages at a time scribbles spontaneously mouthing stops points and gestures puts objects in and takes out of container holds two objects in one hand imitates adult performances turns knobs	

Fine Motor Development, *continued*

4.0 – 5.0 years	5.0 – 6.0 years
makes elaborate structures with blocks copies parquetry design with blocks holds paper with other hand while writing copies a square, triangle, and star folds paper three times traces line within ¼ inch of the original line traces a diamond imitates drawing a square draws a man with 3-6 parts uses both hands independently in building begins to cut more precisely with scissors prints simple words	grips strongly with either hand exhibits mature pencil grip writes and draws with some efficiency copies diamond and rectangle prints name with, then without, a model fastens shoes prints numbers 1-5 draws a person with 6 parts laces shoes and can tie a bow with model
	6.0 – 12.0 years
	colors within the lines cuts and pastes develops sport skills for leisure time develops artistic skills for leisure time

Many sensory and motor skills are involved in the development of oral-motor and feeding skills. The development of oral-motor and feeding skills are interrelated. A delay in one area can affect development in the other.

Oral-Motor and Feeding Skills Development	
0 – 6 months	6 – 12 months
nurses rooting reflex present sucking reflex present phasic bite reflex present sucks or suckles rhythmically using large movements of the jaw and tongue primitive suck-swallow response tongue cups around nipple uses center of lips to hold nipple opens mouth for spoon smiles begins blowing bubbles puts objects in mouth uses coordinated suck pattern, smaller movements of the jaw and tongue with assist by the cheeks demonstrates long sequence of sucking, swallowing, and breathing holds bottle with both hands spoon feeding begins with downward and forward movement of the upper lip and assist of lower lip begins cup drinking using a suckling pattern or mixture of suckling and sucking sucks liquid from a spoon or cup develops munching (i.e., first chews with an up-and-down motion; no rotary chewing or grinding) accepts and swallows smooth and lumpy foods some drooling present	presents a bite-release action (i.e., develops jaw stability, control, and grading required for chewing and biting) presents a sustained bite (i.e., develops the ability to bite through foods like crackers; demonstrating more jaw stability, control, and strength) learns to chew uses both suckling or sucking patterns when drinking removes food from spoon using lips and pulling head back develops cup drinking, may use tongue under cup for stability more coordinated lateral tongue movement true suck-swallow develops tongue developing independence from jaw develops ability to eat table food tongue begins to show more lateralization hand-feeds self, using thumb and first two fingers drool only present when teething bites through a soft cookie brings full spoon to mouth

Oral-Motor and Feeding Skills Development, *continued*	
1.0 – 2.0 years (12 – 24 months)	**2.0 – 3.0 years**
presents controlled sustained bite develops tastes and food preferences primarily takes liquid from a cup may lose liquid while sucking uses cheeks, lips, tongue more actively lips are active during chewing can chew with lips closed intermittently bites on side of cup when drinking, using lips, tongue, and cheeks more actively to control fluid controls degree of mouth opening (jaw grading) uses pronated hand grasp for spoon and fork (i.e., grasps with palm down) dips spoon and fork into food frequently spills from spoon or fork before reaching mouth raises elbow as lifts spoon to mouth cleans lips with tongue presents a graded bite tongue elevation and depression are independent of the jaw gives up bottle drinks through a straw	adequate lip movement during chewing, no loss of liquid or saliva rotary chew fully developed takes controlled bites demonstrates adequate jaw stability for cup drinking learns to eat independently uses supine grasp of spoon and fork, with good rotation of the wrist spills little when eating with spoon holds cup by handle (in adult fashion) tongue fully transfers food laterally
	3.0 – 4.0 years
	spreads with a knife rotary chew fully developed uses fork to stab food
	4.0 – 5.0 years
	eats skillfully with a fork cuts with a knife

Milestones for the Typically-Developing Child
The Source for Down Syndrome

Speech is a motor act that incorporates respiration, phonation, articulation, and resonation to create intelligible communication.

Speech Development	
0 – 6 months produces undifferentiated cry produces sounds on exhalation reflexive sound making produces short, soft nasal sounds produces vowels must actively move body to make sounds develops differentiated cry coos and gurgles produces a variety of vowel and consonant sounds with duration takes turns vocalizing uses loudness and pitch variations produces single syllables babbling begins chuckles and laughs sporadic imitation occurs	words tend to come and go uses gesture with vocalization imitates more consistently uses around 10 words
	1.5 – 2.0 years (18 – 24 months) can imitate whole words produces consonants including bilabials, alveolars, velars, and some stridents uses more words than jargon produces 50-200 words
6 – 12 months sounds produced no longer generated with body movement vocalizes consonants and vowels in play presents a variety of sound combinations babbles using pitch and inflection changes (prosodic contours) uses early-developing consonants (e.g., *p, b, m, n, t, d, k, g, h, wh,* and *sh*) and vowels (e.g., *a, i,* and *u*) imitates intonation patterns begins to jabber begins to use jargon produces first words around 12 months associates sounds he/she makes with an object begins to repeat words heard	**2.0 – 3.0 years** speech intelligibility improves, although prominent substitutions, distortions, and omissions of final consonants still present in words approximately 25% intelligible at 2½ years approximately 80% intelligible at 3 years
	3.0 – 4.0 years produces all vowels and most consonants including bilabials, alveolars, velars, glides, liquids, and some consonant blends intelligibility of connected speech is improved articulator skills become more refined
	4.0 – 5.0 years produces some triple consonant blends very few omissions and substitutions occur by around 4 1/2 years; most consonants are used consistently and accurately intelligibility in conversational speech is good
1.0 – 1.5 years (12 – 18 months) uses all vowels and many consonants in jargon uses several intelligible words first words are context dependent	**5.0 – 7.0 years** uses mature speech

Language is a symbolic system used for communication. Receptive language comprises the comprehension of language. Expressive language comprises the use of language.

Receptive Language Development
0 – 6 months
quiets in response to sound turns to, moves eyes to sound eagerly attends to faces, voices, and gestures learns about world through visual, tactile, and auditory information in environment and caregiver routines gestural communication begins visually tracks responds to own name discriminates between friendly and angry voices gives or shows objects discriminates strangers
6 – 12 months
recognizes family members' names responds with gestures to "Come," "Want Up?," and "Bye-bye" maintains attention to speaker responds to sounds not in visual field recognizes the names of common objects, looks at objects when named comprehends "No" enjoys looking at pictures will give object on request understands commands understands own name
1.0 – 1.5 years (12 – 18 months)
understands 50 words will give two objects requested follows simple one-step commands points to object he/she wants knows three body parts identifies several objects in a picture points to people and toys on request perceives emotions of others possession emerges

Expressive Language Development
0 – 6 months
uses undifferentiated cry makes vegetative, fussing noises, and pleasure sounds differentiated cry develops demonstrates mutual imitation (own sounds) coos, grunts, chuckles, laughs starts babbling uses facial expressions and vocalizations takes turns vocalizing begins to imitate sounds made during interactions with caregiver produces two syllables babbles repetitive syllables
6 – 12 months
vocalizes syllables and syllable combinations imitates environmental sounds and speech sounds imitates duplicated syllables calls to get attention babbling and jargon are present begins to approximate novel sounds first words may be used (context dependent) first words tend to come and go vocalizes to request or command uses three words by 12 months
1.0 – 1.5 years (12 – 18 months)
produces 5-10 words uses mostly nouns vocalizes with gestures answers question "What's this?" recurrence emerges (i.e., asks for "more") asks "What's that?" names 2-7 objects on request uses jargon with real words intermixed

Milestones for the Typically-Developing Child
The Source for Down Syndrome

Receptive Language Development, continued	Expressive Language Development, continued
	uses vocalizations and words to request, command, call attention, establish interaction, greet, protest, and label talks about the present
1.5 – 2.0 years (18 – 24 months)	**1.5 – 2.0 years (18 – 24 months)**

identifies body parts and clothing
follows two-step commands
follows novel commands
comprehends 200-300 words
listens to simple stories and poems over and over
identifies pictures named
responds correctly to *yes/no* questions using a
    head shake
	frequently uses single words
	starts using language as a tool
	jargon peaks; more real words being used
	uses 50-200 words by 24 months
	begins using modifiers (e.g., *more, some*)
	names five or more pictures
	says "No"
	words have a variety of functional and semantic roles
	    (recurrence, existence, non-existence, rejection,
	    denial, agent, object, action, state, location)
	produces successive one-word utterances
	begins to produce two-word utterances
	major vocabulary growth spurt occurs
	frequently uses new words
	use of possessive emerges (e.g., "my hat")
	reproduces animal and environmental sounds
	can talk about things not present
	adjectives, adverbs, and simple verb forms appear
	uses first pronouns
	can imitate and may produce some 3-4 word utterances

2.0 – 2.5 years	**2.0 – 2.5 years**

comprehends approximately 500 words
identifies action and some adjectives in pictures
discriminates between *your* and *my*
understands the concept *one*
understands size concepts
identifies some prepositions (e.g., *on, off, in, out*)
listens to simple stories
identifies objects by use
	uses at least 200 intelligible words
	uses action and adjectives (e.g., colors and size)
	may verbalize toilet needs, but not always effectively
	recites simple nursery rhymes and songs
	names several objects by use
	answers "Where, Who, Whose, What, What are you
	    doing?" and "What do you ___ with" questions
	names one color
	refers to self by pronoun
	produces simple noun or verb phrases
	uses at least two sentence types
	uses negation
	starts to use some prepositions (e.g., *on, in*), present
	    progressive tense, plurals, possessive markers, and
	    the articles *a* and *the*

Receptive Language Development, *continued*	Expressive Language Development, *continued*
	retells daily experiences starts to ask *wh*-questions with the question word at the beginning of the sentence (e.g., "What's that?") says full name uses dialogue in play mean length of utterance approximately 2.0 words
2.5 – 3.0 years	**2.5 – 3.0 years**
comprehends 900-1000 words learns how and why things work identifies parts of an object wants to know "how" and "why" knows own sex comprehends the concepts *up, down, under, beside, big, little, hot, cold* understands quantity concepts *all* and *one* matches colors	uses at least 500 words intelligibly states gender answers *yes/no* questions counts to three verb forms emerging (auxillary "is/am") (e.g., "Bill is sick." "I am hungry.") asks "Why," but may not listen to response uses 3-5 word sentences that are more grammatically correct uses expanded noun phrases can repeat a sentence of 5-7 words starts to ask many questions to gain information uses pronouns *I, me, my, mine, he, she, it* regular past tense emerges adverbs emerging (e.g., *here, there, come here*) begins to use modals (e.g., "I can jump." "Mom will come.") relates simple imaginative tales describes action in books verbalizes toilet needs mean length of utterance approximately 3.1 words
3.0 – 3.5 years	**3.0 – 3.5 years**
comprehends 1000-1200 words has cognitive base for past and future tenses understands the concepts *top, in front of, behind, in back of, hard, soft, rough, smooth, heavy* identifies circle and square matches sets big growth in descriptive vocabulary (e.g., shapes, sizes, colors, textures, spatial relations) begins to use listening skills to learn comprehends complex and compound sentences understands the concept *two*	uses at least 600-1200 words can link two ideas together in a sentence grammar becomes more complex rote counts to 10 asks "is" questions (e.g., "Is that mine?" "Is Daddy home?") fills in last word of a sentence talks about future events and hypothesizes verbalizes intentions third person singular present tense emerges starts to use contracted forms of *is* and modals *won't* and *can't*

Receptive Language Development, *continued*	Expressive Language Development, *continued*
	answers *wh*-questions irregular plurals emerging uses three-word sentences consistently begins to respond correctly to "why" and "how" questions uses language to boss and criticize mean length of utterance approximately 3.5 words
3.5 – 4.0 years	**3.5 – 4.0 years**
comprehends 1500-5000 words aware of perceptual attributes (e.g., color, size, shape, sound) language is used as a tool to think, learn, and imagine completes three-step commands	uses 1500-2000 words uses conjunctions can do simple verbal analogies answers "how much, how long," and "when" questions recognizes 2-3 colors has long, detailed conversations uses the negative *not* combines 4-5 words in a sentence uses complex sentences consistently subordinate clauses emerge begins to use time relational terms (e.g., *now, day, today, tonight*) uses imperatives and emphatics (e.g., "No!," "Stop that!," "I can't.") uses speech to explain, describe, assert, request, and reply mean length of utterance approximately 4.6 words
4.0 – 4.5 years	**4.0 – 4.5 years**
vocabulary continues to grow at a rapid rate understands the concept *three* understands the concepts *between, above, below, bottom, long* understands *if, because, when, why*	uses at least 2000 words defines words in terms of use counts four objects rote counts to 10 repeats four digits inconsistently brags about self (e.g., "I'm a good boy." "I cleaned my plate.") describes what he/she sees language relatively complete in structure and form uses *if* and *so* passive voice emerges (e.g., "The baby was licked by the dog." "The boy was pecked by the bird.") produces 4-7 word complex sentences grammatical errors are less frequent recites the alphabet

Receptive Language Development, *continued*	Expressive Language Development, *continued*
4.5 – 5.0 years	**4.5 – 5.0 years**
comprehends 2500-2800 words identifies four colors on request understands the concepts *light, loud, soft, like, unlike, short* identifies what is missing when several objects are shown, child covers eyes, and one object is taken away classifies by color, form, and use	asks the meaning of words counts 10 objects tells a story in sequence repeats days of the week in sequence uses *first, middle,* and *last* to identify objects in a sequence possessive pronouns emerge comparative "er" emerges produces 5-8 word sentences
5.0 – 6.0 years	**5.0 – 6.0 years**
comprehends 13,000 words understands opposites understands number concepts to 10 knows five alphabet letters identifies penny, nickel, quarter understands the concepts *whole, half, left, right* can identify numbers 1-25 can make shifts in classifying from one form to another (can first clarify by shape, then by size)	counts 12 objects rote counts to 30 names basic colors states similarities and differences uses beginning ordinals identifies numbers 1-10 names days of the week in order uses subordinate clauses (e.g., "I can't go outside because it's raining.") uses all pronouns correctly uses time relational words (e.g., *when, first, next, before, after*) uses comparative adjectives uses irregular verbs correctly uses almost all phrase structures and transformational rules of English recites the alphabet
6.0 – 7.0 years	**6.0 – 7.0 years**
comprehends 20,000-26,000 words understands seasons and attributes knows phone number knows direction or spatial concepts *left* and *right*	can tell address (street and number) names seven capital and lowercase letters has a sight reading vocabulary of at least 10 words uses irregular plurals (e.g., shelf/shelves, sheep/sheep) rote counts to 100 begins to tell time as related to daily routine makes telephone calls

    Milestones for the Typically-Developing Child
The Source for Down Syndrome

Glossary

adenoidectomy	surgical removal of the adenoids
anterior commissure	commissures are nerve fibers that connect structures from one side of the brain to the other; the anterior commissure connects the olfactory bulbs and temporal gyri on both sides of the brain
antihelix/helix	the curved cartilaginous portions of the outer ear
aortic regurgitation	blood flow from the aorta back into the left ventricle of the heart
atlantoaxial instability	an abnormal increase in joint mobility between the first and second cervical vertebrae of the spine; may result in compression of the spinal cord
backward chaining	teaching a task in steps beginning with the last step of the task sequence
cerebellum	the portion of the brain found behind the brainstem; coordinates voluntary muscle activity and is important for muscle tone and equilibrium
cerumen	earwax
collagenous connective tissue	tough fibers that form most of the connective tissue of the body including tendons and ligaments
conductive hearing loss	hearing impairment at the level of the outer or middle ear; often is medically treatable
consolidation	relating and integrating new skills with established skills to promote retention and generalization of learned skills
corpus callosum	white matter that connects the right and left hemispheres of the brain
dendritic spines	the part of a neuron (the basic structural unit of the nervous system) that conveys impulses toward the cell body
epicanthal folds	small skin folds on the inner corners of the eyes; present at birth
external rotation	to rotate outward (e.g., foot, ankle, hip)
faucial pillars	two curved folds of tissue which run between the palate and the tongue at the junction of the oral and pharyngeal cavities; the tonsils are found between the pillars

fissures	deep furrows or grooves
fissuring	furrowing, splitting, or grooving
fistulas	abnormal openings in tissue
forward chaining	teaching a task in steps beginning with the first step of the task sequence
gravitational insecurity	a feeling that one is not safe, stable, or in control of the body when the head is moved in different ways or planes or the feet leave the ground
gyri	convolutions of the cerebral cortex
hematologic dysfunction or disease	a blood disorder or disease
hippocampus	a structure found in the temporal lobe of the brain that is involved in spatial cognition, flexible learning, consolidation of learned skills, and retention of learned skills
Hirschsprung's Disease	a congenital disease of the colon resulting in absence of nerve cells in the rectum and colon that stimulate intestinal mobility; symptoms may include vomiting, diarrhea, and constipation
hyperextension	excessive extension (straightening)
hyperflexibility	excessive flexibility
hypo/hypertelorism	diminished/excessive space between the eyes; narrow or wide-spaced eyes
hypo/hypertonia	diminished/excessive muscle tension or tone
hypoplasia	incomplete or arrested development of tissue
hypoxia	deficiency of oxygen
integration	the organizing, coordinating, combining, and processing of parts (i.e., information from many sources or senses) into a unified whole
intonation contours	the rise and fall of pitch and stress during speaking

The Source for Down Syndrome

joint action routine	routines that involve the same action or related actions around a single theme that is understood by both actors; routines often are commonly known and occur regularly in the child's daily environment with known starting points and ending points, clear role expectations, and response patterns
joint capsules	structures that enclose joints (the connections between bones)
laxity	looseness or slackness
ligamentous laxity	an abnormal increase in elasticity of the ligaments; ligaments join joints, bones, and cartilage
malocclusion	misalignment of the upper and lower teeth
mandible	lower jaw
mandibular angle	the angle of the lower jaw found at the juncture of the body and upward projection of the arm of the mandible
mastoid cells	air cells that are located in the mastoid process of the temporal bone; the temporal bone is found behind and below the outer ear
maxilla	upper jaw
microcephaly	congenital abnormal smallness of the head in relation to the rest of the body
mitral valve prolapse	incomplete closure of the valve between the left atrium and the ventricle of the heart resulting in the backflow of blood
modulation	the brain's regulation of its own activity and consequently the body's activity by controlling and regulating the flow of sensory information; allows the brain to efficiently process sensory information and the individual to respond appropriately and automatically
myelin	protective, fatty sheath that covers nerve fibers
myelination (myelinization)	covering of nerve fibers of the central nervous system by myelin; myelinization of fibers accelerates synaptic connections and makes neural transmissions more precise
nasopharynx	the region of the throat found between the nasal cavity and the soft palate

oblique palpebral fissures	upward slant of the narrow grooves that separate the upper and lower eyelids
occipitofrontal circumference	head circumference
ossicular abnormalities	abnormal shape or positioning of the three small bones of the middle ear that direct sound energy from the tympanic membrane to the inner ear
otitis media	inflammation of the middle ear
palmar crease	a groove across the palm of the hand
pacing board	a board, folder, or paper with a series of dots or other symbols used to visually assist in training rate, stress, breath control, or phrase and sentence production
posterior semicircular canal	one of three tubes in the inner ear that helps in the maintenance of the sense of balance
pronation	lying face down or turning the hand so the palm is down
pulmonary artery hypertension	abnormally high pressure within the pulmonary circulation system
pyloric stenosis	congenital narrowing of the sphincter between the stomach and the small intestines causing a blockage of food into the small intestines
reactivity	the body's level, degree, and speed of response to different stimuli
reduplicated babbling	the production of the same syllable more than once (e.g., "bababa")
registration	how the body acknowledges, reacts, and adjusts to external and internal stimuli
rhinorrhea	free-flowing thin discharge from the nose
scoliosis	lateral curvature of the spine
script	the dialogue, sequential steps, and established roles used in a familiar task, activity, event, or story; the simple text may be accompanied by pictures or written words

152

sensorineural hearing loss	hearing impairment as the result of pathology, damage, or disease in the inner ear or along the auditory nerve pathway from the inner ear to the brainstem
serotonin	a neurotransmitter in the central nervous system
storyboard	the pictured steps of a task, event, activity, or story using photographs, color pictures, or drawings arranged in a sequence of the action to assist the child to complete, retell, or answer questions about the task, event, activity, or story
subglottic stenosis	constriction or narrowing of the airway below the vocal folds
subluxation	partial dislocation
superior temporal gyrus	the superior convolution of the temporal lobe of the brain
synaptic/synapses	the connection between neurons in the brain; the point where communication occurs between one neuron and another
thoracolumbar region	the area of the spine where the thoracic vertebrae join the lumbar vertebrae; the juncture of the upper back and lower back
tonic-clonic convulsions	a type of seizure (i.e., involuntary series of contractions of a group of muscles)
tympanic membrane	the thin membrane that separates the outer ear from the middle ear; the eardrum
tympanometry	a measure used to determine the compliance of the tympanic membrane and middle ear
variegated babbling	the production of differing syllables in a sequence (e.g., "badeeba")
velopharyngeal incompetence (VPI)	inability of the soft palate and the pharyngeal walls to separate the nasal from the oral cavity during speech; results in nasalized speech or an inability to build up air pressure for production of consonant sounds

153

References

Alexander, R. "Oral-Motor and Respiratory-Phonatory Assessment" in Gibbs, E. D. and Teti, D. M. (eds.). *Interdisciplinary Assessment of Infants: A Guide for Early Intervention Professionals.* Baltimore, MD: Paul H. Brookes Publishing Co., 1990.

Ayres, A. J. *Sensory Integration and the Child.* Los Angeles: Western Psychological Services, 1985.

Bailey, D. B. and Woolery, M. *Teaching Infants and Preschoolers with Handicaps.* Columbus, OH: Charles E. Merrill Publishing Co., 1984.

Berube, M. *Life As We Know It.* New York City: Vintage Books, 1996.

Blanche, E. I., Botticelli, T. M., and Hallway, M. K. *Combining Neuro-Developmental Treatment and Sensory Integration Principles.* San Antonio, TX: Therapy Skill Builders, a division of The Psychological Corporation, 1995.

Blacklin, J. and Crais, E. R. "A Treatment Protocol for Young Children At Risk for Severe Expressive Output Disorders." *Seminars in Speech and Language.* New York City: Thieme-Stratton, Inc., Vol. 18, No. 3, 1997.

Brill, M. *Keys to Parenting a Child with Down Syndrome.* Hauppauge, NY: Educational Series, Inc., 1993.

Buckley, S. "Developing the Speech and Language Skills of Teenagers with Down Syndrome." *Down Syndrome Research and Practice*, Vol. 1, No. 2, 1993.

Buckley, S. "Improving the Expressive Language Skills of Teenagers with Down Syndrome." *Down Syndrome Research and Practice*, Vol. 3, No. 3, 1995.

Buckley, S. "Language Development in Children with Down Syndrome: Reasons for Optimism." *Down Syndrome Research and Practice*, Vol. 1, No. 1, 1993.

Butler, K. G. (ed.). "Severe Communication Disorders: Intervention Strategies." *Topics in Language Disorders*, Gaithersburg, MD: Aspen Publications, 1994.

Casby, M. and Ruder, K. "Symbolic Play and Early Language Development in Normal and Mentally Retarded Children." *Journal of Speech and Hearing Research*, Vol. 26, 1983.

Cicchetti, D. and Beeghly, M. *Children with Down Syndrome: A Developmental Perspective.* Cambridge: Cambridge University Press, 1990.

Craighead, N. A. "Strategies for Evaluating and Targeting Pragmatic Behaviors in Young Children." *Seminars in Speech and Language.* New York City: Thieme-Stratton, Inc., Vol. 5, No. 3, 1984.

Crawford, H. "Tangible Symbols." *Advance for Speech-Language Pathologists and Audiologists*, August, 1998.

Cunningham, C. *Understanding Down Syndrome: An Introduction for Parents.* Cambridge, MA: Brookline Books, 1996.

Czesak-Duffy, B. "Metacognitive Approach for the Preverbal Preschooler." *Advance for Speech-Language Pathologists and Audiologists*, April, 1996.

Czesak-Duffy, B. "Oral-Motor Strategies for Modifying Oral Behaviors." *Advance for Speech-Language Pathologists and Audiologists*, March, 1996.

Daly, D. A. *The Source for Stuttering and Cluttering.* East Moline, IL: LinguiSystems, Inc., 1996.

Dell, C. W. *Treating the School Age Stutter.* Memphis, TN: Speech Foundation of America, Publication #14, 1989.

Dmitriev, V. and Oelwein, P. (eds.). *Advances in Down Syndrome.* Seattle: Special Child Publications, 1998.

Doherty, J. "The Effects of Sign Characteristics on Sign Acquisition and Retention: An Integrative Review of the Literature." *Augmentative and Alternative Communication*, Vol. 1, No. 3, 1985.

Duchan, J., Hewitt, L., and Sonnenmeier, R. *Pragmatics from Theory to Practice.* Englewood Cliffs, NJ: Prentice-Hall, Inc., 1994.

Falvey, M. A., McLean, D., and Rosenberg, R. "Transition from School to Adult Life: Communication Strategies." *Topics in Language Disorders,* Vol. 9, No. 1, 1988.

Fisher, M. A. "Social Communication Revision Behaviors in Children with Down Syndrome." *Journal of Childhood Communication Disorders,* Vol. 12, No. 1, 1988.

Frazier, J. B. and Friedman, B. "Swallow Function in Children with Down Syndrome: A Retrospective Study." *Developmental Medicine and Child Neurology,* Vol 38, 1996.

Gard, A., Gilman, L., and Gorman, J. *Speech and Language Development Chart.* Austin, TX: Pro-Ed, 1980.

Gerken, L., and McGregor, K. "An Overview of Prosody and Its Role in Normal and Disordered Child Language." *American Journal of Speech-Language Pathology,* Vol. 7, 1998.

Gibbs, E. and Carswell, L. "Using Total Communication with Young Children with Down Syndrome: A Literature Review and Case Study." *Early Education and Development,* Vol. 2, No. 3, 1991.

Gibson, D. "Down Syndrome and Cognitive Enhancement: Not Like the Others." In Marfo, K. (ed.). *Early Intervention in Transition.* New York City: Praeger, 1991.

Goetz, L., Gee, K., and Sailor, W. "Using a Behavior Chain Interruption Strategy to Teach Communication Skills to Students with Severe Disabilities." *JASH,* Vol. 10, No. 1, 1985.

Gottwald, S. R. and Starkweather, C. W. "Fluency Intervention for Preschoolers and Their Families in the Public Schools." *Language, Speech, and Hearing Services in Schools,* Vol. 26, 1995.

Greenspan, S. and Wiedner, S. *The Child with Special Needs.* Reading, MA: A Merloyd Lawrence Book: Addison-Wesley, 1998.

Halle, J. W. "Arranging the Natural Environment to Occasion Language: Giving Severely Language-Delayed Children Reasons to Communicate." *Seminars in Speech and Language.* New York City: Thieme-Stratton, Inc., Vol 5, No. 3, 1984.

Hanson, M. J. *Teaching the Infant with Down Syndrome.* Austin, TX: Pro-Ed, 1987.

Hodgdon, L. *Visual Strategies for Improving Communication.* Troy, MI: Quirk Roberts Publishing, 1995.

Hodson, B. W. and Paden, E. P. *Targeting Intelligible Speech.* Austin, TX: Pro-Ed, 1991.

Hunt, P. and Goetz, L. "Teaching Spontaneous Communication in Natural Settings Through Interrupted Behavior Chains." *Topics in Language Disorders,* Vol. 9, No. 1, 1988.

Iskowitz, M. "Enhancing Treatment for Severe Speech Disorders." *Advance for Speech-Language Pathologists and Audiologists,* March, 1998.

Iskowitz, M. "Ergonomics in Assistive Technology." *Advance for Speech-Language Pathologists and Audiologists,* August, 1998.

Johnston, S. S. and Reichle, J. "Clinical Forum: Language and Social Skills in the School-Age Population. Designing and Implementing Interventions to Decrease Challenging Behavior." *Language, Speech, and Hearing Services in Schools,* Vol. 24, 1993.

Kavanagh, K. T., Kahane, J. C., and Kordan, B. "Risk and Benefits of Adenotonsillectomy for Children with Down Syndrome." *American Journal of Mental Deficiency,* Vol. 9, No. 1, 1986.

Kleinert, J. "Intervention for Oral Feeding and Vocalization Development with Infants and Toddlers." Short Course, Kentucky Speech-Language-Hearing Association Conference on Communication Disorders, 1997.

Kumin, L. *Communication Skills in Children with Down Syndrome.* Bethesda, MD: Woodbine House, 1994.

Kumin, L., Councill, C., Goodman, M., and Chapman, D. "Down Syndrome: Comprehensive Intervention for Children." *Advance for Speech-Language Pathologists and Audiologists,* October, 1996.

Langley, M. B. and Lombardino, L. J. (eds.). *Neurodevelopmental Strategies for Managing Communication Disorders in Children with Severe Motor Dysfunction.* Austin, TX: Pro-Ed, 1991.

Lott, I. T. and McCoy, E. E. *Down Syndrome: Advances in Medical Care.* New York City: Wiley-Liss, 1992.

MacDonald, J. D. and Carroll, J. Y. "A Social Partnership Model for Assessing Early Communication Development: An Intervention Model for Preconversational Children." *Language, Speech, and Hearing Services in Schools,* Vol. 23, 1992.

MacDonald, J. D. and Carroll, J. Y. "Communicating with Young Children: An Ecological Model for Clinicians, Parents, and Collaborative Professionals." *American Journal of Speech-Language Pathology,* September, 1992.

MacDonald, J. D. and Gillette, Y. "Conversation Engineering: A Pragmatic Approach to Early Social Competence." *Seminars in Speech and Language.* New York City: Thieme-Stratton, Inc., Vol 5, No. 3, 1984.

McLean, J., Yoder, D., and Schiefelbusch, R. *Language Intervention with the Retarded: Developing Strategies.* Baltimore, MD: University Park Press, 1972.

McCormick, L. and Schiefelbush, R. L. *Early Language Intervention.* Columbus: Merrill Publishing Co., 1990.

Marfo, K. (ed.). *Early Intervention in Transition. Current Perspectives on Programs for Handicapped Children.* New York City: Praeger, 1991.

Morris, S. "Developmental Implications for the Management of Feeding Problems in Neurologically-Impaired Infants." *Seminars in Speech and Language.* New York City: Thieme-Stratton, Inc., Vol. 6, No. 4, 1985.

Morris, S. *Pre-speech Assessment Scale.* Clifton, NJ: J. A. Preston Corp., 1982.

Morris, S. *Program Guidelines for Children with Feeding Problems.* Edison, NJ: Childcraft Education Corp., 1977.

Morris, S. E. and Klein, M. *Pre-Feeding Skills.* San Antonio, TX: Therapy Skill Builders, a division of The Psychological Corporation, 1987.

Mosby's Medical, Nursing, and Allied Health Dictionary. St. Louis: The C.V. Mosby Company, 1990.

Mundy, P., Kasari, C., Sigman, M., and Ruskin, E. "Nonverbal Communication and Early Language Acquisition in Children with Down Syndrome and in Normally-Developing Children." *Journal of Speech and Hearing Research,* Vol. 38, No. 1, 1995.

Nadel, L. (ed.). *The Psychobiology of Down Syndrome (Issues in the Biology of Language and Cognition).* Cambridge, MA: MIT Press, 1988.

Nadel, L. and Rosenthal, D. (eds.). *Down Syndrome: Living and Learning in the Community.* New York City: John Wiley and Sons, Inc., 1995.

Newman, I. and Feldman, S. *Readings in Down Syndrome.* Guilford, CT: Special Learning Corp., 1980.

Nicolosi, L., Harryman, E., and Krescheck, J. *Terminology of Communication Disorders.* Baltimore: Williams and Wilkins, 1989.

Nussbaum, S. and Rosenblum, R. *Infant, Toddler, and Preschool Curriculum for Children with Down Syndrome.* Bellmore, NY: Association for Children with Down Syndrome, Inc., 1994.

Oelwein, P. L. *Teaching Reading to Children with Down Syndrome.* Bethesda, MD: Woodbine House, 1995.

Oetter, P. A., Richter, E. W., and Frick, S. M. *M. O. R. E. Integrating the Mouth with Sensory and Postural Functions.* Hugh, MN: PDP Press, 1995.

Page, J. "A Pragmatic Approach to Communication Intervention for Severely and Profoundly Retarded Individuals." Short Course, Kentucky Speech-Language-Hearing Association Conference on Communication Disorders, 1981.

Pecyna Rhyner, P. M. "Graphic Symbol and Speech Training of Young Children with Down Syndrome: Some Preliminary Findings." *Journal of Childhood Communication Disorders,* Vol. 12, No. 1, 1988.

Pentz, A. L. and Moran, M. J. "Voice Disorders in Down Syndrome." *Journal of Childhood Communication Disorders,* Vol. 12, No. 1, 1998.

156 *The Source for Down Syndrome*

Pueschel, S. M. *A Parent's Guide to Down Syndrome: Toward a Brighter Future.* Baltimore: Paul H. Brookes Publishing Co., 1990.

Pueschel, S. M. and Pueschel, J. K. (eds.). *Biomedical Concerns in Persons with Down Syndrome.* Baltimore: Paul H. Brookes Publishing Co, 1992.

Purdy, A. H., Deitz, J. C., and Harris, S. R. "Efficacy of Two Treatment Approaches to Reduce Tongue Protrusion of Children with Down Syndrome." *Developmental Medicine and Child Neurology*, Vol. 29, 1987.

Quinn, P. *Understanding Disability, A Lifespan Approach.* Thousand Oaks, CA: Sage Publications, 1998.

Reichley, M. L. "Selecting Toys for Play with a Purpose." *Advance for Speech-Language Pathologists and Audiologists*, December, 1995.

Rhyner, P. "Graphic Symbol and Speech Training of Young Children with Down Syndrome." *Journal of Communication Disorders*, Vol. 12, No. 1, 1998.

Richard, G. and Hanner, M. A. *Language Processing Remediation.* East Moline, IL: LinguiSystems, Inc., 1987.

Rondal, J. A. and Comblain, A. "Language in Adults with Down Syndrome." *Down Syndrome Research and Practice*, Vol. 4, No. 1, 1996.

Rondal, J. A., Perera, J., Nadel, L., and Comblain, A. (eds.). *Down's Syndrome: Psychological, Psychobiolgical, and Socio-educational Perspectives.* San Diego: Singular Publishing Group, Inc., 1996.

Rosenfeld-Johnson, S. and Manning, D. "Preventing Oral-Motor Problems in Down Syndrome." *Advance for Speech-Language Pathologists and Audiologists*, August, 1997.

Rosin, M. M., Swift, E., Bless, D., and Vetter, D. "Communication Profiles of Adolescents with Down Syndrome." *Journal of Communication Disorders*, Vol. 12, No. 1, 1998.

Roth, F. and Clark, D. "Symbolic Play and Social Participation Abilities of Language Impaired and Normal Developing Children." *Journal of Speech and Hearing Disorders*, Vol. 52, 1987.

Roth, F. P. and Spekman, N. J. "Assessing the Pragmatic Abilities of Children: Part 1. Organizational Framework and Assessment Parameters." *Journal of Speech and Hearing Disorders*, Vol. 49, 1984.

Roth, F. P. and Spekman, N. J. "Assessing the Pragmatic Abilities of Children: Part 2. Guidelines, Considerations, and Specific Evaluation Procedures." *Journal of Speech and Hearing Disorders*, Vol. 49, 1984.

Salzberg, C. and Villani, T. "Speech Training by Parents of Down Syndrome Toddlers: Generalization Across Settings and Instructional Contexts." *American Journal of Mental Deficiency*, Vol. 87, No. 4, 1983.

Scott, A. "Positive Outcomes." *Advance for Speech-Language Pathologists and Audiologists*, August, 1998.

Selikowitz, M. *Down Syndrome: The Facts.* Oxford: Oxford University Press, 1997.

Shriberg, L. and Widder, C. "Speech and Prosody Characteristics of Adults with Mental Retardation." *Journal of Speech and Hearing Research*, Vol. 33, 1990.

Silverman, F. *Communication for the Speechless.* Englewood Cliffs, NJ: Prentice-Hall, Inc., 1980.

Smith, P. and Kleinert, J. (eds.). *Kentucky Systems Change Project: Communication Programming for Students with Severe and Multiple Handicaps.* Kentucky Department of Education, Office of Education for Exceptional Children and the Interdisciplinary Human Development Institute, University of Kentucky, 1991.

Sommers, R. K., Patterson, J. P., and Wildgen, P. L. "Phonology of Down Syndrome Speakers, Ages 13-22." *Journal of Childhood Communication Disorders*, Vol. 12, No. 1, 1998.

Sommers, R. K., Reinhart, R. W., and Sistrunk, D. A. "Traditional Articulation Measures of Down Syndrome Speakers, Ages 13-22." *Journal of Childhood Communication Disorders*, Vol. 12, No. 1, 1998.

Spender, Q., Stein, A., Dennis, J., Reilly, S., Percy, E., and Cave, D. "An Exploration of Feeding Difficulties in Children with Down Syndrome." *Developmental Medicine and Child Neurology*, Vol. 38, 1996.

Stratford, B. and Gunn, P. (eds.). *New Approaches to Down Syndrome*. London: Cassell, 1996.

Stray-Gundersen, K. (ed.). *Babies With Down Syndrome: A New Parents Guide*. Rockville, MD: Woodbine House, 1986.

Stremel-Campbell, K. "The Transition from Prelinguistic to Emergent Language Skills: Assessment and Intervention." Short Course, Kentucky Speech-Language-Hearing Association Conference on Communication Disorders, 1987.

Stoel-Gammon, C. "Normal and Disordered Phonology in Two-Year-Olds." *Topics in Language Disorders*, Vol. II, No. 4, 1991.

Strode, R. M. and Chamberlain, C. E. *Easy Does It for Apraxia and Motor Planning*. East Moline, IL: LinguiSystems, Inc., 1993.

Strode, R. M. and Chamberlain, C. E. *Easy Does It for Articulation: An Oral Motor Approach*. East Moline, IL: LinguiSystems, Inc., 1997.

Swift, E. and Rosin, P. "A Remediation Sequence to Improve Speech Intelligibility for Students with Down Syndrome." *Language, Speech, and Hearing Services in Schools*, Vol. 21, No. 3, 1990.

Tingey, C. *Down Syndrome: A Resource Handbook*. Boston: College Hill Publications, 1988.

Tuchman, D. "Cough, Choke, Sputter: The Evaluation of the Child with Dysfunctional Swallowing." *Dysphagia*, Vol. 3, 1989.

Van-Borsel, J. "An Analysis of the Speech of Five Down's Syndrome Adolescents." *Journal of Communication Disorders*, Vol. 21, No. 5, 1988.

VanDyke, D. C., Lang, D. J., Heide, F., VanDuyne, S., and Soucek, M. J. (eds.). *Clinical Perspectives in the Management of Down Syndrome*. New York City: Springer-Verlag, 1990.

VanDyke, D. C., Mattheis, P., Eberly, S. S., and Williams, J. (eds.). *Topics in Down Syndrome: Medical and Surgical Care for Children with Down Syndrome*. Bethesda, MD: Woodbine House, 1995.

Wadsworth, B. *Piaget's Theory of Cognitive Development*. New York: Longman, Inc., 1971.

Weistuck, L. and Lewis, M. *Language Interaction Intervention Program*. San Antonio, TX: Communication Skill Builders, a division of The Psychological Corporation, 1991.

Weitzman, E. *Learning Language and Loving It*. Toronto, Ontario: The Hanen Center, 1992.

Westby, C. E. "Assessment of Cognitive and Language Abilities Through Play." *Language, Speech, and Hearing Services in Schools*, Vol. II, 1980.

Wilbarger, P. and Wilbarger, J. *Sensory Defensiveness in Children Aged 2-12, An Intervention Guide*. Santa Barbara, CA: Avanti Educational Programs. 1991.

Wishart, J. G. "The Development of Learning Difficulties in Children with Down Syndrome." *Journal of Intellectual Disability Research*, Vol. 37, 1993.

Yoder, P. J., Spruytenburg, H., Edwards, A., and Davies, B. "Effects of Verbal Routine Contexts and Expansions on Gains in the Mean Length of Utterance in Children with Developmental Delays." *Language, Speech, and Hearing Services in Schools*, Vol. 26, No. I, 1995.

Zemlin, W., *Speech and Hearing Science*. Englewood Cliffs, NJ: Prentice Hall, 1988.